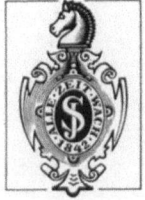

Jean-Noël Bruneton

Ultrasonography of the Neck

With Contributions by C. Balu-Maestro D. Fenart
G. Kalifa J.-F. Moreau F. Normand
J. Poncin J. Santini N. Santini N. Sellier

With 185 Figures

Translated by N. Reed Rameau
Foreword by F. Demard

Springer-Verlag
Berlin Heidelberg New York
London Paris Tokyo

Author

Dr. Jean-Noël Bruneton
Service de Radiologie, Centre Antoine-Lacassagne
36, Voie Romaine, 06054 Nice Cedex, France

Translator

Nancy Reed Rameau
Centre Antoine-Lacassagne
36, Voie Romaine, 06054 Nice Cedex, France

ISBN-13: 978-3-642-71558-7   e-ISBN-13: 978-3-642-71556-3
DOI: 10.1007/978-3-642-71556-3

Library of Congress Cataloging-in-Publication Data.
Bruneton, J.-N. Ultrasonography of the neck. Includes bibliographies and index.
1. Neck-Diseases-Diagnosis. 2. Diagnosis, Ultrasonic. I. Title. [DNLM: 1. Endocrine
Glands-pathology. 2. Lymph Nodes-pathology. 3. Neck-pathology. 4. Ultrasonic
Diagnosis-instrumentation. 5. Ultrasonic Diagnosis-methods.   WE   708 B895u]
RC936.B76   1987   617'.5307'543 86-26021

Typesetting, printing, and binding: Appl, Wemding
2121/3140-543210

Foreword

Owing to the anatomic complexity of the neck and the diversity of pathologic entities affecting it, the cervical region has long been of great semiological interest. Physical examination is an easy means of evaluating the size and origin of a solitary cervical mass, yet valid interpretation can prove difficult when the normal morphology of the neck has been altered; excellent examples are patients with extensive fibrosis or scarring secondary to previous irradiation or surgery. Likewise, physical examination cannot assess the relations of a pathologic process to adjacent structures – e. g., invasion cannot be distinguished from simple displacement – and it is unsuitable for monitoring therapeutic efficacy, such as the response of metastatic nodes to medical management.

Between physical examination, which remains fundamental, and exploratory surgical procedures, which are often the only means of obtaining indispensable anatomic proof for diagnosis, lie a number of recent imaging techniques including computed tomography and magnetic resonance imaging using surface coils that provide invaluable information for the investigation of cervical pathologies. Real-time ultrasonography occupies a privileged position because of its noninvasiveness, rapidity, and reliability, especially when performed by a specially trained examiner.

Jean-Noel Bruneton has methodically explored the multiple applications for ultrasonography of the neck in constant liaison with the Cervicofacial Surgery Department of our institution. As an otorhinolaryngologist specializing in ENT cancers, I wish to thank him for having so clearly presented his experience in this particularly instructive book, which should prove to be a constant reference for the reader in the appraisal of cervical pathologies.

François Demard, MD
Director, Centre Antoine-Lacassagne, Nice

The authors wish to thank Christine Rostagni,
Françoise Fein, and Bernard Fontaine for their assistance
in the preparation of this book.

Contents

2   *Thyroid Gland*
         J.-N. Bruneton and F. Normand 22

List of Contributors

Catherine Balu-Maestro
Service de Radiologie, Centre Antoine-Lacassagne
36, Voie Romaine, 06054 Nice Cedex, France

Jean-Noel Bruneton
Service de Radiologie, Centre Antoine-Lacassagne
36, Voie Romaine, 06054 Nice Cedex, France

Denis Fenart
Service de Radiologie, Centre Antoine-Lacassagne
36, Voie Romaine, 06054 Nice Cedex, France

Gabriel Kalifa
Service de Radiologie, Hôpital Saint Vincent de Paul
74, Avenue Denfert Rochereau, 75674 Paris Cedex 14, France

Jean-François Moreau
Service de Radiologie, Hôpital Boucicaut
78, Rue de la Convention, 75015 Paris, France

Frank Normand
Service de Radiologie, Centre Antoine-Lacassagne
36, Voie Romaine, 06054 Nice Cedex, France

Jocelyne Poncin
Service de Radiologie, Hôpital Saint Vincent de Paul
74, Avenue Denfert Rochereau, 75674 Paris Cedex 14, France

José Santini
Service de Chirurgie Cervicofaciale, Centre Antoine-Lacassagne
36, Voie Romaine, 06054 Nice Cedex, France

Nicole Santini
Service de Radiologie, Centre Antoine-Lacassagne
36, Voie Romaine, 06054 Nice Cedex, France

Nicolas Sellier
Service de Radiologie, Hôpital Saint Vincent de Paul
74, Avenue Denfert Rochereau, 75674 Paris Cedex 14, France

1 Medical Ultrasound Equipment, Examination Technique, and Ultrasonography of the Normal Neck

J.-N. Bruneton, N. Santini, and J. Santini

For convenience, cervical ultrasound can be artificially divided into studies of the anteromedial or visceral compartment, and explorations of the lateral neck. The anteromedial neck was one of the first anatomic regions to benefit from contact ultrasound scanning, and the earliest publications on thyroid sonography date back more than 10 years. Owing to the difficulty in exploring the lateral neck by contact scanning, examination of this region has benefited greatly from the introduction of high frequency, real-time equipment. Thus, the ultrasonic characteristics of nodal and salivary gland pathologies have been defined only recently. This chapter deals successively with ultrasound equipment and technological advances, examination techniques, and the ultrasonic appearance of the normal structures of the neck.

1.1 Equipment

Whereas in the early 1980s many real-time ultrasound units were still not equipped with a high frequency transducer (at least 7.5 MHz), this significant technological advance is currently widely available. The emphasis in this section is thus placed on real-time equipment; contact scanning is described merely for the sake of completeness.

1.1.1 Real-Time Ultrasound Equipment

Real-time ultrasonography, which provides a dynamic and permanent image (permanence is actually due to persistence of vision), has numerous advantages:

- the short time required for examination allows use of ultrasonography (US) for almost all patients, although the quality of the study is variable
- the dynamic nature of ultrasonography allows evaluation of the mobile structures of the neck such as vessels, which are highly pulsatile in certain patients; functional assessment of swallowing prevents confusion of the esophagus with a pathological lesion
- examiner training is facilitated by easy-to-use transducers

In fact, the basic problem with real-time ultrasonography of the neck is the need for complete familiarity with cervical anatomy. Its only real drawback is the limited field of view (triangular or trapezoidal with sector transducers, rectangular with linear transducers). The suitability of sector transducers has been questioned for cervical investigations, and particularly for thyroid studies, as visualization of an entire enlarged lobe on a single sagittal scan can be difficult. Although this can be considered a disadvantage from an iconographic viewpoint, it is actually an advantage for the sonographer: the small size of sector transducers makes examination easy to perform regardless of the contour of the neck and the patient's ability to maintain cervical hyperextension (Leopold 1980). The rapidity and efficacy of real-time sector scanning, as well as the limited value of a sonogram for the uninitiated, mean that the examination should be performed whenever possible by a specialized physician. Electronically focused resolution systems and phased array transducers represent two of the most recent developments in the field of medical ultrasonics, but this new equipment has not yet proven inherently superior to traditional high-frequency transducers.

In addition to film and paper records of sonographic images, videotapes are useful for functional assessment of the tongue. Static imaging of selected frames allows analysis of the oral phase of swallowing and is a valuable adjunct for the evaluation of speech. It appears to be unnecessary in other circumstances.

1.1.2 Contact Scanning

Contact scanning, the oldest sonographic technique, relies on manual movement of the transducer; the quality of this static examination thus depends heavily on the sonographer. The only potential cause of motion artifacts in the anteromedial neck is a hyperpulsatile carotid artery. The higher resolution of contact transducers than real-time equipment, at least up until the past few years, partially explains the satisfactory results of thyroid contact scanning. Today, however, the only generally recognized indication remaining for contact scanning is the dimensional workup of a large goiter unsuited for real-time exploration, the ultimate aim being comparison of scans obtained over a period of time.

1.1.3 Other Techniques

All four ultrasonic applications described below are based on real-time procedures.

1.1.3.1 Intraoperative Ultrasonography

Intraoperative ultrasonography is of limited value for cervical pathologies. It utilizes the same transducers as intraoperative abdominal ultrasonography, with preference given to linear probes. When indicated, this technique is described in the chapters on individual neck structures, but two potential uses merit particular comment:

- Ultrasonic localization of enlarged parathyroid glands is a sensitive complementary procedure that can shorten the duration of surgery;
- Except when a specific search is being made for cancer, surgical exploration of the entire thyroid gland appears unnecessary if the lobe contralateral to a thyroid lesion is sonographically normal. Intraoperative ultra-

sonography appears especially advisable if a deep lesion smaller than 5 mm, visualized on a previous sonogram, is not detected by intraoperative palpation. US-directed biopsy of such nodules is recommended.

There are actually relatively few indications for intraoperative cervical ultrasonography, and none of our personal studies concerning the cervical lymph nodes and the salivary glands revealed any major benefit from the technique that would warrant its use during cervicofacial surgery.

1.1.3.2 Ultrasonographic Tissue Characterization

In view of the prevalence of benign tumors of the neck, and especially those affecting the thyroid gland, development of a means that would facilitate therapeutic decisions, i. e., surgical vs medical management, represents a much sought-after goal. For the thyroid gland in particular, the most sensitive noninvasive means for prospective differentiation of benign and malignant pathologies seems to be a technique based on the recording of digitized radiofrequency signals (Benson et al. 1983). This procedure has not yet become routine as the sophisticated equipment required is currently available only at certain specialized institutions.

1.1.3.3 Pulsed Doppler Ultrasound

The use of pulsed Doppler techniques for cervical explorations is restricted to analysis of a lesion's blood supply. For the present, at least, this procedure does not seem capable of differentiating between benign and malignant lesions, and especially not those of the thyroid gland. Moreover, both adenomas and adenocarcinomas may be either hypo- or hypervascularized. Pulsed Doppler is utilized primarily to determine whether or not a lesion is hypervascularized. It has diagnostic implications as hypervascularized lesions should only be punctured with caution, using a fine needle, whereas hypovascularized lesions can be examined at low risk using a coarse needle or microbiopsy procedure. This aid in selection of the biopsy procedure for cytology studies should increase the technique's sensitivity for cervical lesions.

1.1.3.4 Ultrasound-Directed Aspiration Biopsy

This technique was somewhat neglected until recently as palpation combined with cytology seemed sufficient for diagnosis and therapeutic decisions. In actuality, the frequency of sub-clinical neck lesions underscores the need for a reliable biopsy procedure, such as exists for deep visceral lesions, on which therapeutic decisions can be based. The literature contains few reports of complications attributable to cervical puncture for either diagnostic purposes (obtaining cell samples or tissue microfragments) or, less frequently, for therapeutic purposes (ablating parathyroid tumors for example). Although sector transducers have been utilized, preference is usually given to the type of bar transducer employed for intraoperative studies (Rizzatto et al. 1985). Roughened Teflon-coated needles are reportedly the easiest type to visualize with ultrasound (McGahan and Walter 1985).

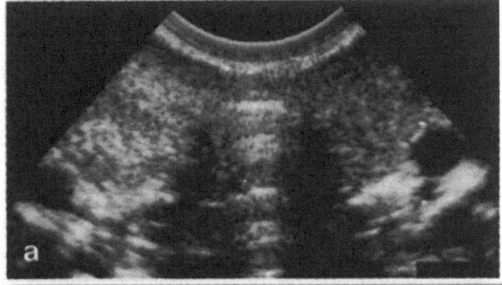

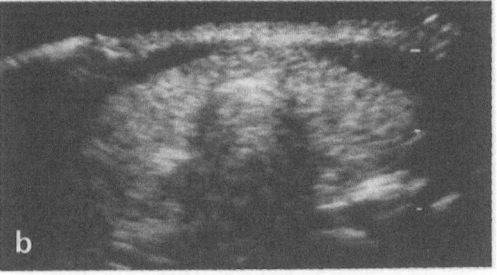

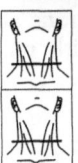 **Fig. 1.1a, b.** Transverse scan of the antero-medial neck showing both thyroid lobes, with (**a**) and without (**b**) a water bath. The larynx and trachea, forming the upper airway, occupy a medial position and contain reverberation echoes (**a**)

1.1.4 Transducer Frequency

When ultrasound exploration of the anterior neck and especially the thyroid gland was first introduced, 3.5 MHz contact transducers were considered satisfactory. Currently, real-time examinations can easily be performed with transducers of at least 7.5 MHz. Use of a water bath or Reston interface is mandatory with 5 MHz transducers to obtain acceptable results. In practice, the transducer used depends on the projected type of examination; as emphasized by the following examples, it must be selected as a function of both the patient and the pathology.

The first example concerns exploration of the thyroid gland, which may appear normal with a 7.5 MHz transducer, even though it contains a small superficial lesion. In these cases examination must be completed using a water bath or Reston interface.

The second example also concerns the thyroid. Both 7.5 and 10 MHz transducers can diagnose thyroid tumors, but if the lesion is malignant

and requires thyroidectomy, possibly followed by neck irradiation, ulterior searches for disease recurrence may not be satisfactory with 7.5 or 10 MHz probes. Cutaneous thickening secondary to irradiation may necessitate the use of a 5 MHz transducer.

In addition to these factors related to the nature of the lesion and the patient's medical history, ultrasound transmission varies from one individual to another, independently of the amount of subcutaneous tissue. Furthermore, exploration of the entire tongue up to the level of the tonsil using a submental approach generally requires a 5 MHz transducer; a higher frequency transducer can only be employed in certain limited favorable cases.

To summarize, most real-time cervical explorations are performed with a 7.5 MHz transducer; depending on the circumstances a lower frequency or, on the contrary, a water bath or Reston interface (allowing better analysis of superficial structures) may be advisable (Fig. 1.1).

1.2 Examination Technique

The rapidity of real-time ultrasonography of the neck and the value of histological examination of biopsy material facilitate and justify adoption of a comprehensive US approach. As an example, detection of a thyroid or parathyroid nodule should be followed by US exploration of all of the cervical node regions for associated nodal involvement. Diagnosis can then be oriented towards a malignant process. Likewise, discovery of a parotid nodule justifies exploration of the other salivary glands due to the possibility of systemic disease.

This section is limited to the general features of the technique; the anatomic landmarks for US studies are given in italics in Sect. 1.3. For purposes of clarity, explorations of the anteromedial and lateral compartments have been dealt with separately, even though both regions are explored during the same session with real-time equipment.

1.2.1 Exploration of the Anteromedial Neck

1.2.1.1 Thyroid Gland: Supine Position

In the ideal position, the patient lies supine with a pad under the shoulders, the neck hyperextended, and the chin elevated, thereby making the maximum possible cervical area accessible to examination. This is the preferred position for exploration of the lower neck region, especially when a mediastinal extension of the thyroid is suspected.

1.2.1.2 Thyroid Gland: Other Positions

When the supine position is not feasible, several modified examination positions can be employed: low back pain can be relieved by having the patient bend his knees, and patients with cervical arthrosis can be examined after the head is slightly rotated away from the side of interest. When hyperextension is impossible, and this is the case for many elderly patients and individuals with cardiac or respiratory insufficiency, examination may be performed with the patient sitting down or with the examination table tilted only slightly. Real-time sec-

tor scanners guarantee optimum patient comfort and an examination of good quality. Real-time examination also permits localization of mediastinal thyroid tissue, as such structures rise into view when the patient swallows. In a similar manner, identification of the esophagus by its peristaltic activity prevents confusion with an enlarged parathyroid gland. Both coronal and sagittal scans are necessary.

1.2.1.3 Tongue

Exploration of the tongue requires an examination position similar to that for the thyroid gland, with the patient's neck hyperextended and the chin raised whenever possible. A line drawn from the middle of the chin down to the laryngeal cartilages facilitates delineation of the midline of the tongue; this point is of considerable importance as the location of a lingual cancer relative to the midline influences the therapeutic approach.

Patients with cancer of the tongue cannot always be examined with the neck hyperextended, but real-time equipment and especially sector transducers almost always allow satisfactory evaluation of both tumor size and the extent of spread towards the midline and in depth. Having the patient keep his mouth filled with water is unnecessary for examination of a cancer of the tongue or tonsil, but it can be useful when videotaping the oral phase of swallowing. Study of the oral phase of swallowing relies essentially on sagittal scans, while both sagittal and transverse scans are indispensable for cancers of the tongue.

1.2.2 Exploration of the Lateral Neck

Whereas contact scanners allowed satisfactory examination of the anteromedial neck, the recent progress in exploration of the lateral cervical regions is due to the introduction of real-time equipment. Acceptable evaluation of the superficial neck regions, and especially of superficial nodal masses and spinal chain nodes, requires use of a water bath or Reston interface in addition to a high frequency transducer.

1.2.2.1 Superficial Cervical Nodes

The superficial cervical nodes are usually examined in real-time after localization of the common carotid artery and the internal jugular vein. Transverse scans obtained between these two important landmarks, starting from the lower neck and working up, allow accurate evaluation of the relationship of a nodal mass to the carotid artery or internal jugular vein at any point. US can generally visualize the jugular chain nodes lying anterior to the carotid artery and the internal jugular vein, and the spinal chain nodes posterior to these two landmarks (cf. Sect.1.3.5). Despite their limited diagnostic value, sagittal scans are useful from an iconographic standpoint; for example, both thrombosis of the internal jugular vein and the node responsible for compression can be visualized on the same scan.

1.2.2.2 Submandibular Gland

Use of a submaxillary approach permits visualization of the entire submandibular gland.

1.2.2.3 Parotid Gland

The parotid gland is usually examined by transverse scans obtained using a subauricular approach between the mandible anteriorly and the mastoid process posteriorly (the distance between these two bones is variable). Sagittal scans are helpful in the rare instances that they succeed in visualizing the intraparotid vessels. Analysis of the venous and arterial involvement of a tumor necessitates exploration along the vascular axes, i.e., scans sagittal to the gland itself. Examination of the parotid gland must be completed by exploration of the masseter muscle located anteriorly; although the normal parotid duct cannot be visualized, anomalies can be detected by use of a water bath.

1.2.3 Special Circumstances

Ultrasonographic examination of children must be performed rapidly, and thus in real-time, us-

ing the same technique as for adults. Pediatric patients are best examined by an experienced sonographer capable of completing exploration in the shortest possible time.

The gain setting used depends on the sonographer and available equipment, but an examination is best started with a low gain that can be increased progressively according to the requirements of the structures examined.

In addition to recording lesion images on film and photographic prints, the use of *surgical maps* or charts is a helpful means of exchanging sonographic data (cf, Chaps. 2 and 5). Such maps allow the physician who initially requested the sonogram to readily evaluate the extent of any lesions and, if the patient has been managed medically, to assess any resultant modifications.

1.2.4 Pitfalls and Technical Artifacts

The rare problems encountered in ultrasonography of the neck are more often due to the inexperience of the sonographer than to patient-related factors.

Reverberation echoes can occur when a water bath or Reston interface is used, or even simply when the patient has a highly adipose neck. They are easily recognized as they lie parallel to the planes of contact (skin-ultrasound and water-ultrasound). They are easily eliminated by modifying the transducer–skin distance, for example, by pressing the transducer down slightly harder against the water bath or Reston interface. In practice, during real-time examinations, the sonographer solves this problem spontaneously by moving the transducer whenever a parasite image appears.

Inappropriate selection of the transducer and the gain can be considered a "beginner's error." The gain should be adjusted so that the entire thyroid gland appears sonographically homogeneous. Transducer selection depends on the desired examination results, and a decrease in image quality is only normal when a 7.5 MHz transducer is replaced by a 5 MHz probe. However, 5 MHz transducers allow better analysis of deep structures, such as are required for examinations of the tongue.

Limited physical mobility in a patient always results in an examination of subnormal quality as fewer anatomic structures can be localized and evaluated.

Other patient-related factors affecting examination quality include *obesity,* which may manifest sonographically as stratifications in the superficial neck regions, and the consequences of *previous radiotherapy.* Patients with radiation-induced cutaneous thickening must be examined with a 5 MHz transducer; the images will not be of the best quality, but a 7.5 MHz transducer is unsuitable. In addition to the sequelae of extensive burns, *cervical scars* can hinder ultrasonographic examination to varying degrees. Real-time examination allows satisfactory exploration of patients with a lobo-isthmectomy scar. By contrast, the sonograms obtained of patients who have undergone severely mutilating surgery (parathyroid operations in some cases) or surgery completed by radiotherapy are often unsatisfactory.

Very few pitfalls and artifacts are actually encountered with ultrasound studies of the neck. Except in certain particular circumstances (severe arthrosis, previous surgery, or high dose irradiation), technical problems are easily solved. The major problem for the sonographer is familiarity with the anatomy of the neck.

1.3 Ultrasonography of the Normal Neck

This section describes in succession the normal ultrasonographic anatomy of the thyroid gland, the parathyroid glands, the salivary glands, the tongue, and the superficial cervical nodes. The high resolution of state-of-the-art sonographic equipment allows recognition of anatomic structures of little or no practical interest, yet certain structures of real pathological importance cannot be visualized (for example, the excretory ducts of the parotid and submandibular glands). The potential applications and limitations of ultrasonography have therefore been indicated along with the anatomic features for each structure. Anatomic details are given in normal typescript and ultrasonographic data in italics.

1.3.1 *Thyroid Gland*

1.3.1.1 *Anatomy*

The thyroid is an endocrine gland located in the infrahyoid region of the neck; its concave posterior surface is applied against the antero-lateral surfaces of the larynx and the first tracheal rings. The thyroid gland consists of two lateral lobes connected by a median structure, the isthmus, at the junction of the lower and middle thirds.

The lateral lobes are shaped like triangular pyramids with their summit directed upward; they present three surfaces (anterior, medial, posterior), three borders (anterior, posterolateral, posteromedial), and two extremities (a narrow apex cephalad and a thicker base caudad). Average lobe dimensions are: height 4–6 cm, width and thickness 1–2 cm. Ultrasound allows volumetric analysis of the thyroid lobes. Each lobe can be considered a spheroid whose volume (v) is given by:

$$v = \frac{\pi}{6} \times \text{height} \times \text{width} \times \text{depth}$$

The average volume of a thyroid lobe has been estimated at between 12 and 40 cm³ (Hegedus et al. 1982). The volume in cm³ generally corresponds to the weight in grams. The sensitivity of volumetric computations can be increased to nearly 95% by determining the surface area from contiguous transverse scans (Tannahil et al. 1978).

The base of each thyroid lobe is directed inferiorly to within 1 or 2 cm of the sternum, but this position varies from one individual to another. The base of one or both lobes may be located even lower, at the level of the cervicothoracic junction; this renders examination more difficult and requires considerable hyperextension of the neck for proper exploration. In other patients, the base of one or both lobes lies higher up in the neck, 4–5 cm above the sternum; this is relatively frequent in young women.

Finally, the thyroid lobes are often slightly asymmetrical, with the right lobe tending to be larger than the left. Moreover, lobes are not always both located at the same level in the neck, and this can create a false impression of asymmetry on transverse scans. The isthmus varies from 1 to 2 cm in height. The pyramidal lobe (Lalouette's pyramid) is an inconstant conical structure projecting upward from the isthmus, either along the midline or off to one side.

Thyroid tissue has a highly uniform, solid US pattern consisting of a dense agglomerate of very fine small echoes of equal size (Fig. 1.2). In certain cases high frequency transducers can visualize intrathyroid vessels as small rounded structures on scans perpendicular to the axis of the vessel or as small linear structures on scans parallel to the axis of the vessel. In most cases such images represent small dilated veins. The isthmus is always well visualized by ultrasound, especially when a high frequency transducer or water bath is used (Fig. 1.3). By contrast, the normal pyramidal lobe can never be seen owing to its small anteroposterior diameter (1–2 cm when this lobe exists). The sonographic appearance of the thyroid gland is often less homogeneous in elderly individuals.

1.3.1.2 Anterior and Posteromedial Relations (Poncin-Viateau and Hassan 1985)

The anterior relations of the thyroid gland are common to the lateral lobes, the isthmus, and the parathyroid glands (Fig. 1.4).

The superficial covering consists of skin, the platysma, and subcutaneous tissue. Sonographically, this covering corresponds to a thin, highly echogenic band averaging 2 mm in thickness; exact thickness depends on the person's weight. A stratified appearance is fairly common in obese individuals.

The *investing layer of the deep cervical fascia* forms a sheath encasing the sternocleidomastoid muscles laterally. These muscles are always well visualized by ultrasonography; although variable in thickness, they can be recognized by their elongated shape anterior to the lateral aspect of the thyroid lobes. The anteroinferior extremity of these muscles is located to one side of the midline. This investing layer of the cervical fascia contains the anterior jugular veins. *Regardless of their thickness, the sternocleidomastoid muscles have a solid US pattern that is markedly less echogenic than the normal thyroid gland. This difference is of practical use for comparative analysis of the thyroid gland, in particular in cases of diffuse thyroid hy-*

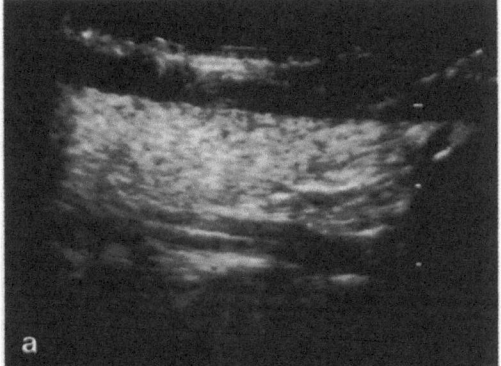

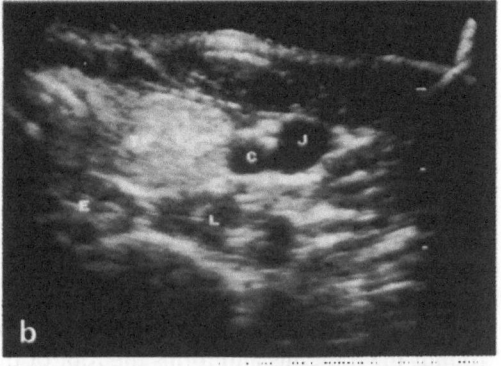

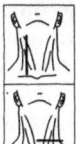

Fig. 1.2 a, b. Normal thyroid lobe as seen on a sagittal scan (**a**) and a transverse scan (**b**). *C,* common carotid artery; *J,* internal jugular vein; *L,* longus colli muscle; *E,* esophagus; *T,* thyroid

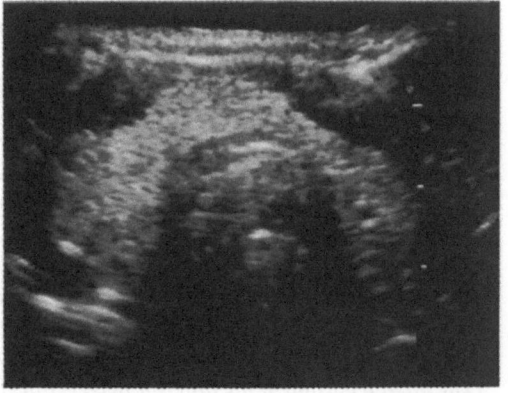

Fig. 1.3. Nonpathological homogeneous enlargement of the thyroid isthmus (transverse scan obtained with a water bath). The superficial cervical muscles anterior and lateral to the medial aspect of the thyroid lobes are less echogenic than the thyroid gland

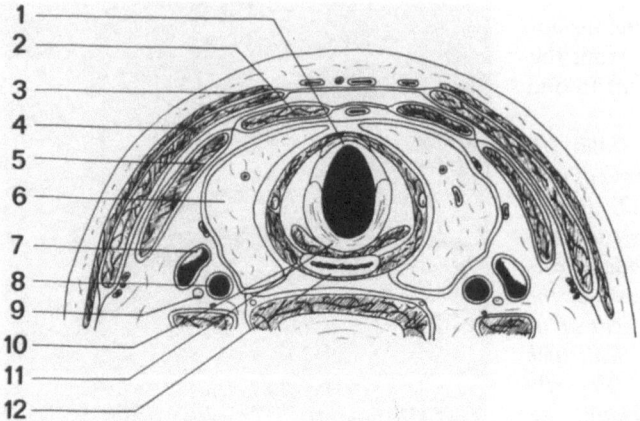

Fig. 1.4. Anatomy of the anterior neck. *1*, trachea; *2*, sternocleidohyoid muscle; *3*, platysma; *4*, sternocleidomastoid muscle; *5*, omohyoid muscle; *6*, thyroid gland; *7*, internal jugular vein; *8*, common carotid artery; *9*, vagus nerve; *10*, inferior pharyngeal constrictor muscle; *11*, cricoid cartilage; *12*, esophagus

poechogenicity such as occur with thyroiditis. The anterior jugular veins cannot be visualized by ultrasound unless the internal jugular vein is thrombosed.

In addition to enclosing the sternocleidomastoid muscles, this investing fascial layer surrounds the trapezius and forms the roof of the posterior cervical triangle, enclosing the omohyoid muscle; it also covers the infrahyoid muscles, forming the roof of the anterior triangle. *This muscular layer can be examined with high frequency transducers, and is particularly well visualized in patients with a muscular neck. The US image, similar to that of the sternocleidomastoid muscles, corresponds to a hypoechogenic band anterior and lateral to the thyroid lobes.*

Posteromedial relations of the thyroid gland involve the thyroid lobes, the gastrointestinal tract, and the major neurovascular bundle.

The medial surface of the thyroid lobes is related, from front to back, to the upper airway (larynx and trachea) and to the pharynx and esophagus. *These anatomic structures can be identified on sonograms as a very dense echogenic line, corresponding to the anterior wall, next to an acoustic shadow representing the air-filled cavity. The medial portion of the anterior neck is thus inaccessible to US because of this acoustic artifact behind the thyroid gland, but this does not interfere with exploration of the entire thyroid gland.*

The gastrointestinal tract is represented by the inferior constrictor muscle of the pharynx and the esophagus. The esophagus crosses over the trachea on the left side, and can be seen at the posteromedial border of the left thyroid lobe. *The esophagus is visualized sonographically as a semicircular bull's-eye with a hyperechogenic center and less echogenic contours; the hyperechogenic area corresponds to the esophageal lumen and the less echogenic peripheral structure to the esophageal wall. This image is inconstant and visible to varying degrees depending on the subject. Particular care must be taken not to mistake an esophageal deviation on the left side of the neck for a cervical mass, and in particular a parathyroid gland. The mobility of this structure can be examined in real-time studies by having the patient swallow (Fig. 1.5).*

The **posterior surface of the thyroid lobes** is related to the cervical vertebrae, the longus colli muscle, and the major neurovascular bundle. *From back to front are visualized sonographically the dense interface of the anterior surface of the cervical vertebrae, then the transversally elongated longus colli muscle which is only slightly echogenic. The longus colli muscle may be shaped either like a trapezoid with its largest base directed outwards, or like a triangle with its apex directed medially. This muscle is bounded anteriorly by the interface formed by the deep layer of the cervical fascia. In contrast to those muscles related to the thyroid gland anteriorly, the longus colli muscle is an important anatomic landmark for cervical ultrasonography, yet may be difficult or impossible to visualize in individuals with muscular atrophy (elderly patients or those with a neurologic pathology).*

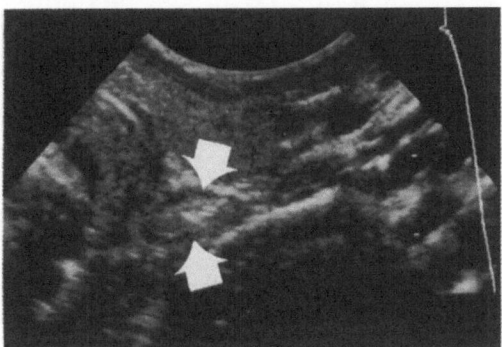

Fig. 1.5. Transverse scan of the esophagus *(arrows)* in a lateral position in the left side of the neck, posterior to the thyroid gland

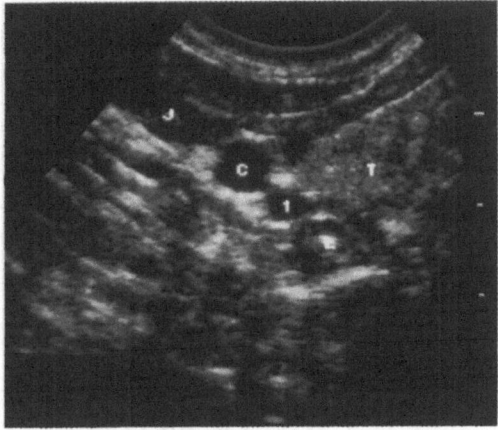

Fig. 1.6 Transverse scan of the thyroid showing the inferior thyroid pedicle (*I*). C, common carotid artery; *J*, internal jugular vein; *L*, longus colli muscle; *T*, thyroid gland

The **major neurovascular bundle** comprises the common carotid artery (with the internal carotid artery and external carotid artery located cephalad), the internal jugular vein (lateral to the artery and more or less spontaneously visible), and the vagus nerve. *The sheath enclosing the major neurovascular bundle cannot be seen sonographically, but the common carotid artery is always recognizable on transverse scans as an anechoic circle with a solid circumference. An atheromatous or hyperpulsatile carotid artery can interfere with exploration of small adjacent neck structures. On transverse scans, a sectional view of the internal jugular vein is obtained external to the carotid artery. As the internal jugular vein is not always spontaneously visible, a Valsalva maneuver must be performed systematically: the resultant venous dilatation allows satisfactory examination. The vagus nerve lies in the posterior angle of the common carotid artery and the internal jugular vein and cannot be visualized by ultrasonography.*

The **posteromedial border of the thyroid lobes** is intimately related to the recurrent laryngeal nerve and the inferior thyroid pedicle. *The recurrent nerve cannot be demonstrated by ultrasound. The inferior thyroid pedicle crosses over the posterior surface of the thyroid lobe and divides at the junction of the lower and middle thirds of the lobe; on sonograms it corresponds to a thin, hypoechogenic zone lying transversally at the level of the lower third of the posterior surface of the thyroid lobe. The pulsatile nature of this pedicle can be evidenced in certain patients by real-time examination (Fig. 1.6).*

1.3.1.3 Blood Supply (Fig. 1.7)

The **arterial supply** is provided by the terminal branches of the thyroid arteries:

- The *superior thyroid artery* is the main vascular structure. This paired, symmetrical artery arises from the external carotid artery and divides at the superior pole of the thyroid gland into three branches (superficial, medial, posterior). The medial branch anastomoses with its homologue from the contralateral superior thyroid artery; the posterior branch anastomoses with its homologue from the inferior thyroid artery.
- The *inferior thyroid artery* is also paired and symmetrical. It arises from the subclavian artery and divides at the junction of the lower and middle thirds of the posterior border of the thyroid lobe into three branches (medial, inferior, and posterior). The inferior branch forms the subisthmic anastomosis; the posterior branch forms the longitudinal retrolobar anastomosis with the homolateral branch of the superior thyroid artery. Contrary to the superior thyroid artery, the inferior thyroid artery is absent on rare occasions.
- the *lowest thyroid artery* is an inconstant branch that runs upward from the aortic arch or the innominate trunk to the isthmus.

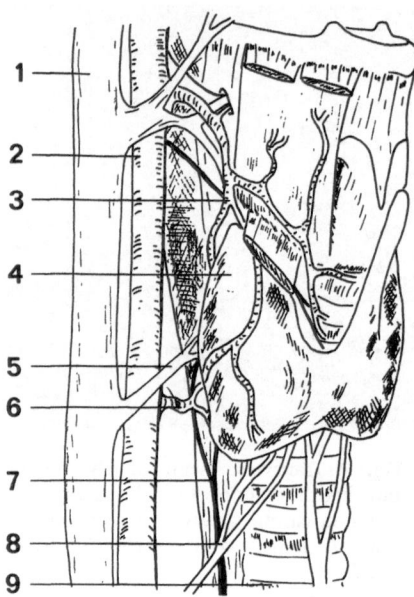

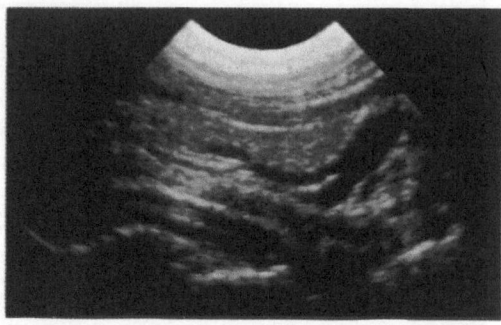

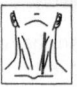
Fig. 1.8. Dilated, intrathyroid veins, without jugular vein thrombosis, or thyroid dysfunction (no Graves' disease)

Fig. 1.7. Thyroid chart indicating the gland's blood supply. *1*, internal jugular vein; *2*, common carotid artery; *3*, superior thyroid artery; *4*, thyroid gland; *5*, middle thyroid vein; *6*, inferior thyroid artery; *7*, recurrent laryngeal nerve; *8*, inferior thyroid vein; *9*, trachea

While the superior thyroid artery represents the major blood supply of the thyroid gland and is easily visualized, it is of little practical use for ultrasound studies. By contrast, the inferior thyroid artery, with the adjacent venous trunk, is a particularly helpful landmark for localizing a normally positioned inferior parathyroid gland.

The **venous drainage** of the thyroid gland begins from a dense subcapsular plexus, then divides into three trunks on each side:

- the *superior* thyroid vein is paired and a satellite of the artery; it drains into the internal jugular vein (thyrolinguofacial trunk)
- the *inferior* thyroid veins form several trunks, anastomosed together, and drain into the left innominate vein
- the *middle* thyroid vein is inconstant; transverse on a normal size lobe, this vein may lie in an anteroposterior direction against a hypertrophic gland and thus complicate surgical hemostasis

Sonographically, the thyroid veins may be easier to visualize than the arteries, especially if the in-

ternal jugular vein is thrombosed. However, the veins can be visualized in those rare instances of intrathyroid varices without jugular vein thrombosis (Fig. 1.8).

The **lymphatic vessels** located at the periphery of the thyroid vesicles (follicles) form a subcapsular network giving rise to both medial and lateral collecting trunks. These collecting trunks are generally satellites of the thyroid veins. The two major lymph node groups are:

- the lateral and anterior nodes of the internal jugular chain
- the pretracheal nodes and the recurrent laryngeal nerve nodes, which drain parallel to the innominate trunks and to the origin of the superior vena cava.

The existence of direct connections, without any nodal relays, between the thyroid lymphatics and the mucosal plexus of the trachea explains the tracheal involvement observed with certain thyroid cancers.

The normal lymph nodes cannot be visualized by ultrasonography. However, systematic exploration of the lateral neck regions is essential during thyroid workups as detection of subclinical adenopathies may orient the etiological diagnosis towards malignancy. From a practical viewpoint, ultrasonography suffices for exploration of the internal jugular chain, but the pretracheal nodes and drainage system of the superior mediastinum require examination by computed tomography.

To conclude, the normal thyroid lobe is oval or triangular on longitudinal US scans. The anterior relations are muscular; the posterior relations vary with transducer inclination. When the transducer is inclined inward, the usual landmark is the longus colli muscle; the inferior vascular thyroid pedicle, when it exists, can also be seen. A left-sided bull's-eye image that moves when the patient swallows should be recognized as a laterally located esophagus.

The internal carotid artery and the internal jugular vein can be identified by inclining the transducer outward.

The triangular shape of the thyroid lobes can be distinguished on transverse scans, but the central area is inaccessible because of the acoustic vacuum formed by the larynx and trachea. Use of a water bath allows visualization of the isthmus, anterior to the larynx and trachea.

1.3.2 Parathyroid Glands

Most individuals have four parathyroid glands lying between the thyroid gland and its capsule. They are usually located on the medial dorsal aspect of each thyroid lobe, between the common carotid artery and deep jugular vein laterally, the tracheoesophageal groove medially, and the longus colli muscle posteriorly.

The average normal parathyroid gland weighs 20–40 mg, and averages 3–6 mm in length, 2–4 mm in width, and 1–3 mm in thickness. Although structures of these dimensions can generally be identified by ultrasonography, the normal parathyroid glands cannot, because their echostructure is indistinguishable from that of the thyroid gland and the adjacent subcutaneous tissue (Sample et al. 1979). This limitation of ultrasound for the localization of the normal parathyroid glands also applies to intraoperative usage. As emphasized by Moreau and Carlier-Conrads (1984), the problem is not gland size, but rather the absence of any difference in echogenicity between the thyroid gland and the normal parathyroid glands.

Topographically, the parathyroid glands are grouped around the terminal branches of the inferior thyroid artery; Bismuth et al. (1975) situated the superior parathyroid glands above this artery, in a posterior position (latero- or retroesophageal). The inferior parathyroid glands are located below the point at which the inferior thyroid artery enters the thyroid space; the lower glands are usually more anterior than the

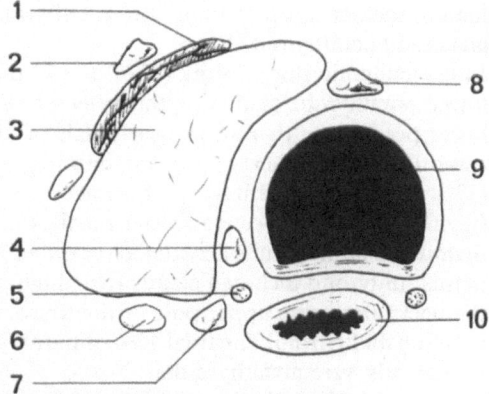

Fig. 1.9. Possible parathyroid positions (excluding mediastinal sites). *1,* sternothyroid muscle; *2,* external parathyroids; *3,* thyroid gland; *4,* intratracheothyroid parathyroids; *5,* right recurrent laryngeal nerve; *6,* retrolobar parathyroids (usual location); *7,* retrorecurrent nerve parathyroids; *8,* external parathyroids; *9,* trachea; *10,* esophagus

upper glands, and are applied against the lower end of the thyroid lobes (Fig. 1.9).

1.3.2.1 Variations in Location

The embryology of the parathyroid glands explains the possible variations in their position and number. The parathyroid glands can be recognized on the 8–9 mm embryo as localized bilateral anlages arising from the third and fourth branchial pouches. When the third pouch separates from the pharynx, the lower gland (parathyroid III), derived from the third branchial pouch, forms a bilobular complex with the thymic lobe (thymus III). As the heart descends into the thorax, it pulls along both the thymus III and the parathyroid III. In the 18 mm embryo the parathyroid III usually lies at the level of the lower pole of the thyroid lobe, and it remains in this position after dissociating from the thymus. In certain individuals, however, one or both inferior glands fail to separate from the thymus and descend lower than usual; such parathyroid glands may be found low in the neck, in the anterior mediastinum, or in the pericardium. In other cases, premature separation (developmental arrest) of the thymus and the parathyroid III can leave the latter high in the neck, cephalad to both the thyroid gland and parathyroid IV.

In his anatomic study, Wang (1976) found the lower parathyroid glands at the level of the lower pole of the thyroid in nearly half of all cases (42%). Another 41% were intrathymic (39% could be visualized in the lower neck (thymic tongue), 2% were in the mediastinal thymus). Ectopic glands accounted for only 2% in this study, and included glands lying high in the neck, above the upper pole of the thyroid, or in the midthyroid. The final 15% of parathyroid glands were juxtathyroidal.

Parathyroid IV (the superior parathyroid glands) forms a bilobular complex with the lateral thyroid. When the thyroid fuses together, parathyroid IV separates from it, acquiring its definitive position as the superior parathyroid immediately above the junction of the inferior thyroid artery and the recurrent laryngeal nerve. As parathyroid IV has a more medial position and is associated with the medial structures of the neck, it migrates less than parathyroid III; its position is therefore more constant, at least in height. For Wang (1976) parathyroid IV is located at the cricothyroid junction or a juxtacricoidal site in slightly over three-quarters of all cases (77%); less often (22%), parathyroid IV may be found behind the superior pole of the thyroid. Only 1% of Wang's cases had parathyroid IV in a retropharyngeal or retroesophageal site.

Overall, Wang (1976) found only 3% of parathyroid glands to occupy mediastinal, retropharyngeal, or retroesophageal sites, and an average incidence of 5% can reasonably be proposed for anatomic variations (Castleman and Roth 1978).

1.3.2.2 Variations in Number

Various anatomic studies place the number of parathyroid glands between two and eight, although the most frequent number is four (two superior, two inferior). The incidence of supernumerary glands varies from 2%–7%; this developmental anomaly may correspond either to multiple gland divisions during embryologic descent (divided glands) or to parathyroid remnants deposited along the path of descent (rudimentary glands).

Awareness of these possible variations in the number and location of the parathyroid glands is essential for recognizing an intrathyroid parathyroid adenoma or the presence of more than four nodular masses due to hyperparathyroidism affecting supernumerary glands.

1.3.2.3 Blood Supply

While an understanding of the blood supply of the parathyroids has no practical applications in ultrasonography, the unquestionable utility of angiographic findings warrants a brief anatomic review.

Arterial Supply. Each parathyroid gland receives a terminal arteriole, and the blood supply is usually assured by the branches of the inferior thyroid artery and, accessorily, by the superior thyroid arteries. Ectopic glands in the neck and mediastinum are generally fed by the inferior thyroid artery, although in certain cases the supply is from a mediastinal artery (internal mammary artery or thymic artery) (Bismuth et al. 1975).

Venous Drainage. The parathyroid glands are drained by three pairs of veins arising from an anastomotic plexus: the inferior thyroid veins drain either separately or after fusion into the innominate venous trunk, while the middle and superior thyroid veins drain into the internal jugular vein. In fact, there are numerous possible variations; ectopic glands in particular may drain into the inferior thyroid veins or into the internal mammary, thymic, or azygos veins.

Familiarity with vessel anatomy is essential for investigations relying on phlebography, as when step samples are required for radioimmunoassay of serum parathyroid hormone. Venous sampling is a helpful procedure for localizing ectopic parathyroid glands that have escaped surgical detection (cf. Chap. 3).

1.3.3 Salivary Glands

1.3.3.1 Parotid Gland

The parotid gland lies in the posterior portion of the prestyloid (parapharyngeal) space; together with the facial nerve, the external carotid artery, the confluent venous plexus, and lymphatic structures, the parotid is enclosed by a fascial, ligamentous, and membranous capsule.

Boundaries and Relations of the Parotid Space

Superficial Relations. From superficial to deep, the structures revealed by physical and US examination include the skin, the fat pad, the subcutaneous tissue containing the extracapsular lymph nodes, and the superficial cervical fascia which encloses the sternocleidomastoid muscle posteriorly and inserts into the masseteric fascia anteriorly (Figs. 1.10 and 1.11). *This generally thin capsule is depicted sonographically as a strongly echogenic band between the ascending ramus of the mandible anteriorly and the mastoid bone posteriorly.*

Anterior Relations. The anterior boundary of the parotid space is formed by bone and muscle: the posterior border of the ascending ramus of the mandible is surrounded by the masseter muscle laterally, and the medial projection extends along the internal pterygoid muscle and the interpterygoid fascia. *Owing to the acoustic shadow of the mandible, only the masseter muscle is visible sonographically; use of*

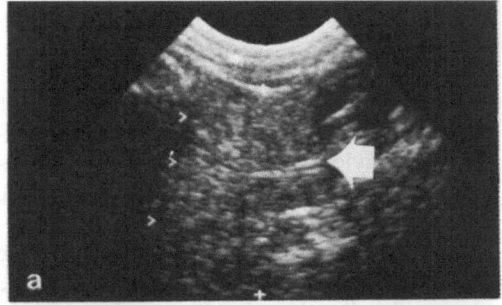
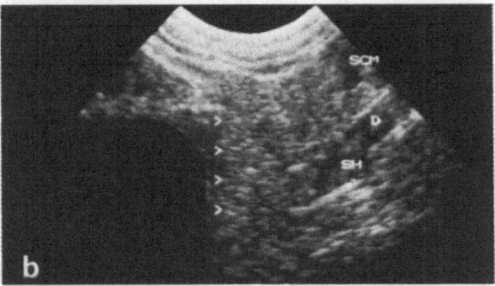
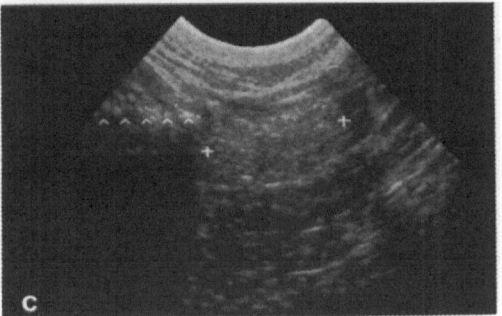

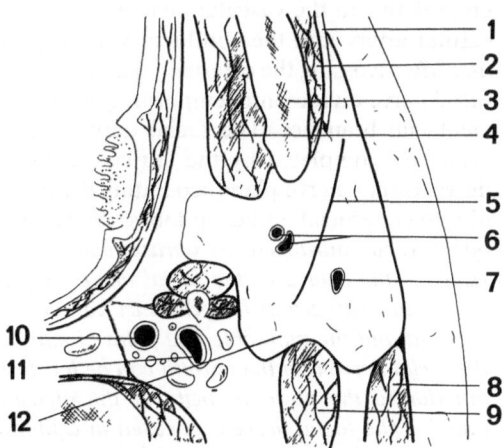

Fig. 1.10. Diagram of a transverse scan of the parotid space. *1,* parotid duct; *2,* masseter muscle; *3,* mandible; *4,* internal pterygoid muscle; *5,* facial nerve; *6,* external carotid artery and vein; *7,* external jugular vein; *8,* sternocleidomastoid muscle; *9,* digastric muscle; *10,* internal carotid artery; *11,* internal jugular vein; *12,* parotid gland

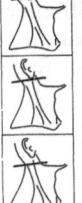

Fig. 1.11 a–c. Transverse scans of the parotid gland, from top to bottom. **a** Upper transverse scan showing the potential point of entry of the facial nerve *(arrow);* anteriorly, acoustic shadow corresponding to the mandible *(small arrows);* 29 mm between the two *crosses.* **b** Middle transverse scan (2 cm below **a**). The sternocleidomastoid *(SCM),* digastric *(D),* and sternohyoid *(SH)* muscles form the posterior boundary of the parotid space. Anteriorly, acoustic shadow of the mandible *(small arrows).* **c** Lower transverse scan (Zem below **b**) of the inferior pole of the parotid (20 mm between the two crosses). Acoustic shadow of the mandible *(small arrows).* **c** Lower transverse scan (2 cm below **b**) of the inferior pole of the parotid (20 mm between the two *crosses*). Acoustic shadow of the mandible *(small arrows)*

a water bath or Reston interface is required in certain cases.

Posterior Relations. The posterior surface of the parotid space is formed by the lateral portion of the styloid diaphragm between the anterior belly of the sternocleidomastoid muscle and the stylomandibular ligament. This posterior wall separates the parotid space from the retrostyloid space. *This wall is not always visible sonographically when the distance between the mastoid bone and the mandible is short. When it can be seen, it manifests as a hypoechogenic zone with bosselated contours. The various muscular and ligamentous structures (anterior belly of the sternocleidomastoid muscle, stylomandibular ligament) can be visualized on transverse scans.*

Medial Relations. The medial surface of the parotid space is closed off by a thin fascial strip that descends into the anterior subparotid space (paratonsillar region). Over 50% of the population present with a pharyngeal parotid extension that is intimately related to the pharynx. *US examination of this medial extension is nearly impossible, and CT or magnetic resonance imaging are indicated for evaluation of this region.*

Inferior Relations. A fascial extension separates the parotid from the submandibular gland. At this level, the parotid descends 1 cm below the inferior aspect of the mandible; certain individuals have a parotid extension that can extend up to 4 cm below the angle of the mandible.

Contents of the Parotid Space

The *parotid gland* is the largest and most posterior of the salivary glands. Irregularly shaped like an inverted pyramid, the parotid is bounded anteriorly by the ascending ramus of the mandible and posteriorly by the mastoid process. The parotid presents a variable number of extensions, the most important being the pharyngeal extension. The excretory duct of the parotid (Stensen's duct) has a diameter of 3 mm; the bayonetlike course of this duct proceeds around the masseter muscle before opening out in the mouth, opposite the second upper molar. *The parotid gland has a sonogra-*

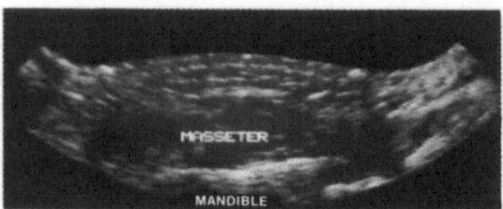

Fig. 1.12. Transverse scan through the masseter region (7.5 MHz transducer with water bath): the superficial cervical fascia, the masseter muscle, and the mandible are visualized. The parotid duct cannot be seen

phically homogeneous appearance, consisting of fine, dense echoes that are more echogenic than the structures forming the boundaries of the parotid space. US cannot visualize the deep portion of the parotid or its medial extensions, and particularly not extensions behind the mandible. The normal parotid duct cannot be seen on sonograms, not even using a high frequency transducer, water bath, or Reston interface, which habitually allow detailed analysis of superficial structures (Fig. 1.12).

The *facial nerve* emerges from the skull through the stylomastoid foramen and enters the superior deep portion of the parotid gland. Up until this point it is the most medial of the parotid space structures; here it becomes the most lateral relative to the vascular elements (external carotid artery and the confluent venous plexus). After crossing the external jugular vein, the facial nerve divides into temporofacial and cervicofacial branches. The facial nerve and its branches, completed by the auriculotemporal nerve, form a nerve plane separating the parotid into superficial and deep lobes. *Neither preoperative nor intraoperative ultrasonography can visualize the course of the facial nerve. In patients with a sufficiently long distance between the mastoid and the mandible, the point of entry of the facial nerve into the parotid can be localized anterior to the posterior belly of the digastric muscle. The facial nerve is encased in a fibrous sheath that is easily recognized by the surgeon, but is indistinguishable sonographically from the surrounding glandular tissue. Nevertheless, the facial nerve is usually located 2.5-3 cm from the reference point on the skin; this anatomic notion is sufficiently reliable for localization of parotid tumors lateral to the facial nerve.*

The *external carotid artery* forms a groove as it penetrates the posterior surface of the gland. This artery terminates 4 cm above the angle of the mandible and divides into the maxillary artery and the superficial temporal artery. *In this case as well, the quality of ultrasound examination depends on the distance between the mastoid and the mandible. When the distance is sufficient, the external carotid artery may be visible at all points in the parotid space as a pulsatile, tubular structure (Fig. 1.13).*

The *venous plane* lies lateral to the external carotid artery, immediately behind the nerve plane formed by the dividing branches of the facial nerve. In most individuals, the veins unite within the parotid gland and drain primarily into the external jugular vein and the internal jugular system. In other cases, the veins unite anterior to the gland, and there are only one or two veins instead of a plexus. *The venous plexus is not visible sonographically. By contrast, the venous plane can be visualized if one or two veins ensure drainage, if necessary by performing a Valsalva maneuver. The nerve plane lies less than 10 mm lateral to the veins, a fact which is of considerable importance when evaluating tumoral pathologies (Fig. 1.14).*

The *parotid lymph nodes* consist of three groups: the suprafascial and subfascial extraglandular parotid, and the intraparotid nodes, which predominate around the venous plane. These nodes receive lymph from the scalp, the temple, and the upper face, and drain into the internal jugular vein chain. *The normal lymph nodes cannot be visualized by US.*

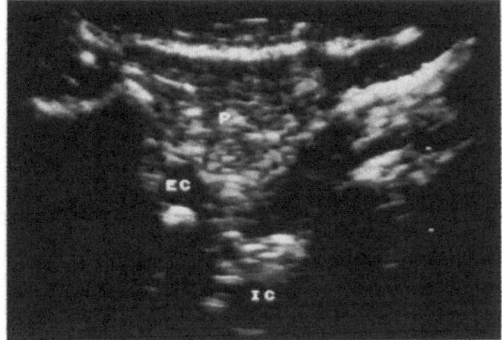

Fig. 1.13. Arterial relations of the parotid gland as seen on a transverse scan. *EC,* external carotid artery; *IC,* internal carotid artery; *P,* parotid gland

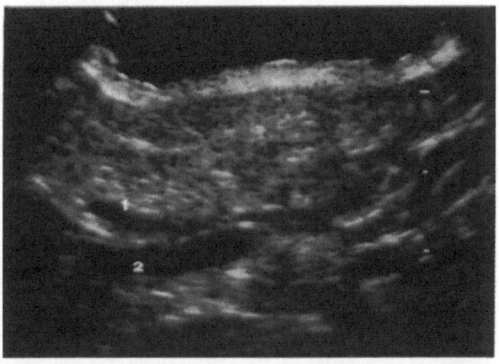

Fig. 1.14. Sagittal scan of the parotid gland: vascular relations. *1,* venous plane; *2,* arterial plane

1.3.3.2 Submandibular Gland

The submandibular region lies below the lingual and sublingual regions, anterior to the bicarotid and carotid regions, in the lateral portion of the space between the hyoid bone and the inferior border of the ramus of the mandible. The importance of this region is due more to the presence of the lymphatic collecting channels of the tongue than to the submandibular gland itself.

Boundaries of the Submandibular Space (Fig. 1.15)

The superolateral boundary is formed by the mandible and the superficial plane below. The medial boundary is divided into two levels by the hyoid bone and is bounded by the subhyoid, pharyngeal, and lingual muscles. Anteriorly, the submandibular space is bounded by the mylohyoid muscle. Posteriorly, the superior part of the submandibular space is related to the elements of the parotid space.

Contents of the Submandibular Space

The submandibular gland is an almond-shaped body oriented obliquely downward, anteriorly,

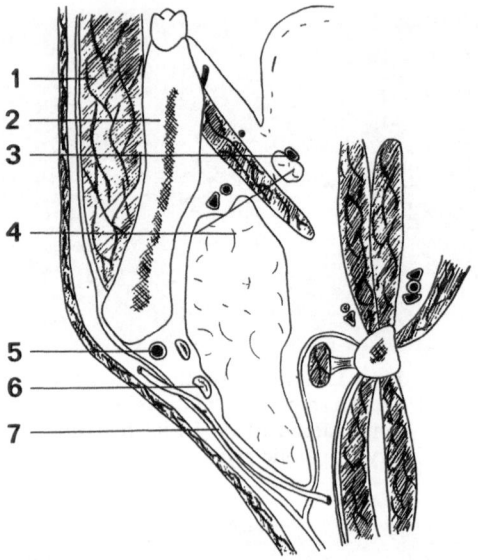

Fig. 1.15. Diagram of a frontal scan of the submandibular space. *1,* masseter muscle; *2,* mandible; *3,* submandibular duct; *4,* submandibular gland and anterior extension; *5,* facial artery; *6,* submaxillary node; *7,* facial vein

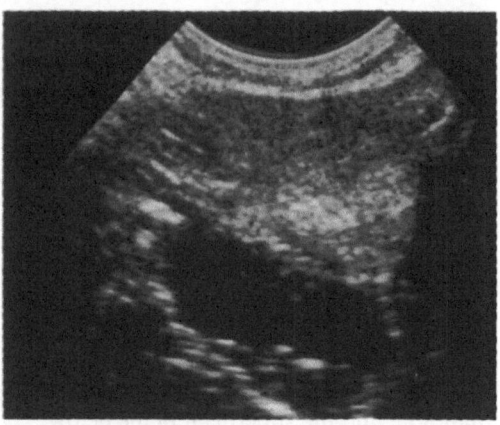

 Fig. 1.16. Ultrasonographic appearance of the normal submandibular gland

and medially. The submandibular duct (Wharton's duct) emerges from the gland's inferior surface and terminates at the side of the frenulum of the tongue. *The entire submandibular gland can be seen by US; its appearance is similar to that of the parotid (Fig. 1.16).* The submandibular space also contains the facial artery

and vein, the lingual nerve, and especially the submaxillary lymph nodes that drain the greater portion of the tongue and the floor of the mouth. *The facial vein can be localized by US. The facial artery is harder to see because it is usually smaller than the vein. The normal submaxillary lymph nodes are not visible on sonograms.*

1.3.4 Tongue

The tongue projects into the oral cavity and occupies the midportion of the floor of the mouth. Roughly oval-shaped, with a large posterior extremity, the tongue is flattened from top to bottom. This muscular organ is characterized by its great mobility.

The body of the tongue presents two surfaces, two margins, and a tip (or apex) (Fig. 1.17). The *dorsal surface* (dorsum) is divided into oral (anterior) and pharyngeal (posterior) parts by an inverted V-shaped groove (the sulcus terminalis) whose point is the foramen cecum. The dorsal surface of the oral tongue is related to the palate and may present a shallow median groove extending from the foramen cecum to the tip of the tongue. The dorsal surface of the pharyngeal tongue is nearly vertical and faces the pharynx.

Sonographic examination of the dorsal surface using a submental approach is only possible when the tongue is "at rest," lying low in the mouth. The pharyngeal portion of the dorsal surface is almost always visible whereas the anterior portion of the oral tongue can prove hard to visualize; the tip of the tongue is especially hard to discern because of the nearly constant interface created by air between the tip and the floor of the mouth. Analysis of the dorsal surface of the tongue can be improved by having the patient keep his mouth filled with water during examination (Shawker et al. 1985).

The *inferior surface* of the tongue presents a median fold of mucous membrane or frenulum, two large longitudinal masses corresponding to the genioglossus muscles, and two lateral fimbriated folds which separate the muscular masses from the lateral borders of the tongue. *The nearly constant presence of saliva in the mouth places the inferior surface of the tongue in intimate contact with the floor of the mouth: this*

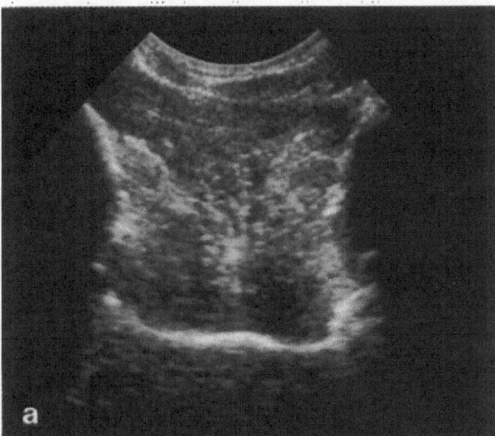

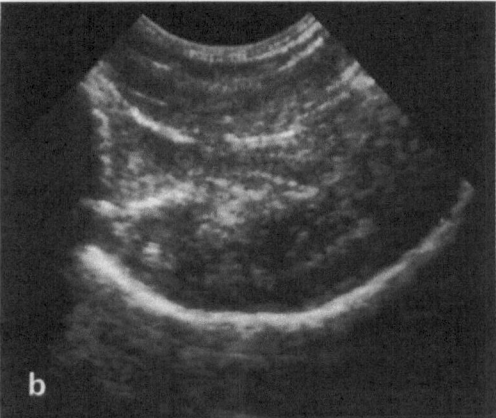

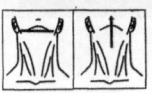

Fig. 1.17. a Transverse and **b** sagittal scans of the normal tongue

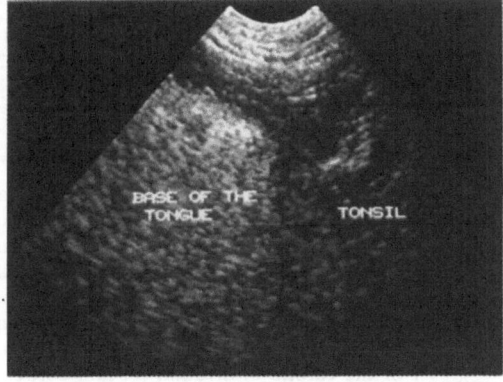

Fig. 1.18. Tonsilloglossal sulcus

allows US analysis of the lingual musculature by a submental approach. Evaluation of tumors on the floor of the mouth requires cooperation on the part of the patient in keeping his tongue raised up during examination. When this is impossible, the patient should be asked to keep his mouth filled with water; this allows elements belonging to the floor of the mouth to be distinguished from those belonging to the inferior surface of the tongue.

There are 17 different **lingual muscles,** all of which are paired except for the superior longitudinal muscle. The largest of these muscles is the genioglossus, a wide, fan-shaped muscle overlying the geniohyoid muscle. *The genioglossus muscle is the easiest to demonstrate sonographically because of its large size and typical fan shape; when a 7.5 MHz transducer is suitable, this muscle is readily visualized; lower frequency probes are incapable of discerning these anatomic details.*

The muscles of the tongue are divided into intrinsic and extrinsic groups. In addition to the genioglossus, the extrinsic muscles include the hypoglossus, the chondroglossus, the styloglossus, and the palatoglossus. The intrinsic group comprises the superior and inferior longitudinal muscles, the transverse muscle, and the vertical muscle.

Two other muscles must also be familiar to the sonographer because these superficial elements are always visible during submental US of the tongue. These are the mylohyoid (most superficial) and geniohyoid muscles. In practice, submental studies visualize well the mylohyoid, geniohyoid, and genioglossis muscles. Exploration starting at the chin and proceeding toward the hyoid region analyzes the lingual musculature and also the tongue's relations with the floor of the mouth and the palatine tonsils posteriorly. Easier to demonstrate in children than in adults, the palatine tonsils are separated from the base of the tongue by the glossotonsillar sulcus; a space-occupying mass in this sulcus during examination for tonsillar cancer indicates spread to the base of the tongue (Bruneton et al. 1986) (Fig. 1.18).

*The **arterial blood supply** is ensured by the dorsal lingual artery and the ranine artery; the **venous blood** drains essentially into the lingual or ranine veins. Familiarity with the **lymphatic drainage** of the tongue is more important for an understanding of the mode of spread of carcinomas. The lymph vessels of the tip of the tongue drain into the submental nodes; all of the other lymph vessels drain into the submandibular, internal jugular, and above all anterior nodes of the internal jugular chain, which must be examined from the digastric muscle to the omohyoid muscle. *Although the normal lymph nodes are not visible sonographically, all US examinations of the tongue must be completed by exploration of the submaxillary and jugulocarotid regions.*

1.3.5 Superficial Cervical Lymph Nodes

As stated previously, the normal lymph nodes cannot be visualized by US because their pattern is indistinguishable from that of the surrounding subcutaneous tissue. For the same reason, even a large lipomatous node (essentially seen in axillary and inguinal sites) cannot be recognized by ultrasound, although it may be visible radiologically. Nevertheless, familiarity with the normal anatomy and features of the cervical nodes is essential for thorough nodal workup of ENT cancers. This anatomic review is followed by a discussion of suggested means of increasing the usefulness of US findings for both the surgeon

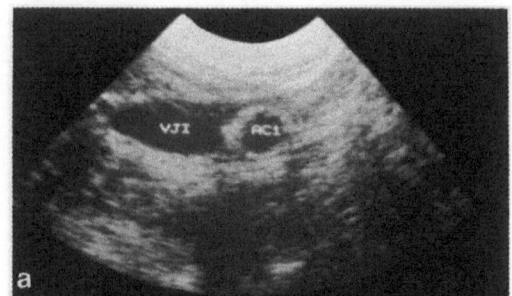
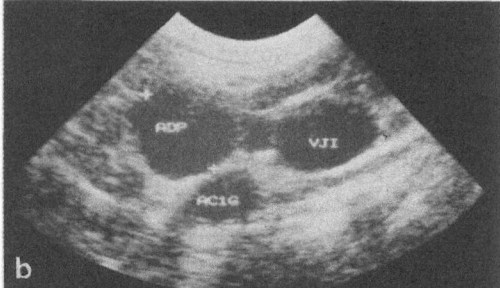
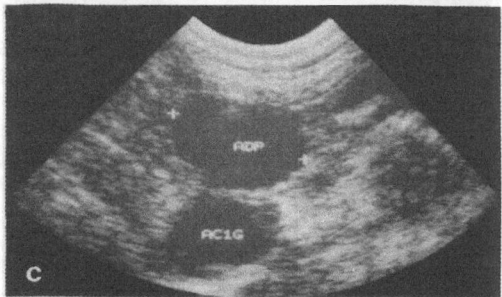
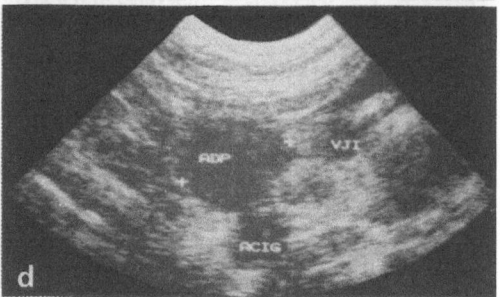

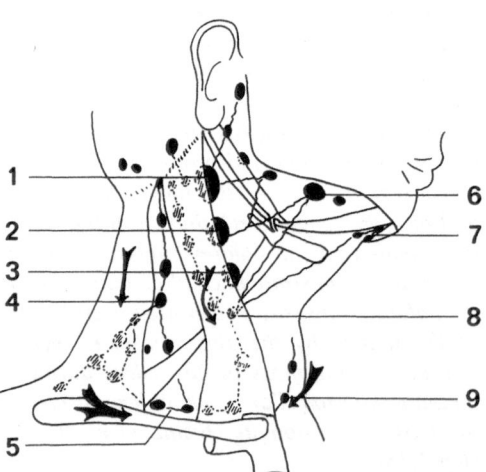

Fig. 1.19. The cervical lymphatic triangle. *1*, principal node of Kuttner; *2*, midjugular node; *3*, lower jugular node; *4*, spinal accessory chain; *5*, transverse cervical chain; *6*, submaxillary nodes; *7*, submental nodes; *8*, internal jugular vein chain; *9*, anterior jugular vein chain

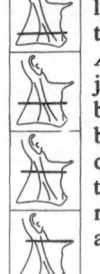

Fig. 1.20a–d. Exploration of the cervical lymph node areas by transverse scans (metastatic nodes of ENT cancer). **a** Low scan. *AC1*, common carotid artery; *VJI*, internal jugular vein. **b** Scan 2 cm above the carotid bifurcation. *ADP*, metastatic node (14 mm between the two *crosses*). **c** Scan at the level of the carotid bifurcation (20 mm between the two *crosses*). **d** Scan 2 cm above the carotid bifurcation. *ACIG*, left internal carotid artery; (17 mm between the two *crosses*)

and the histopathologist (Bruneton et al. 1984). The lymph nodes of the head and neck regions lie between the investing layer of the deep cervical fascia and the prevertebral fascia. Rouvière (1932) classed them into 10 main groups that can be divided into three main chains: the pericervical collar, the deep cervical nodes, and the accessory chains (Fig. 1.19 and 1.20).

1.3.5.1 Pericervical Collar

The pericervical collar consists of nodal groups located at the junction of the head with the neck, from the tip of the chin to the nape of the neck. These groups include:

- the *occipital nodes,* which drain the lymphatics of the nape of the neck and the scalp
- the *retroauricular (mastoid) nodes,* which generally undergo adipose involution in the adult; these nodes drain the parietal scalp, part of the auricle of the ear, and the external auditory canal
- the *parotid nodes* comprise three subgroups: the suprafascial extraglandular, the subfascial extraglandular, and the intraglandular (intraparotid) nodes; these drain the parotid gland, the middle and external ear, and part of the face and scalp
- the *submandibular nodes* include the preglandular and retroglandular nodes (located at the anterior and posterior poles of the gland), the prevascular nodes (the most constant group, which runs along the facial artery), and the intracapsular nodes (lying within the submandibular gland). These four subgroups drain an area including the lips, the cheeks, the upper and lower gums, the tongue, the soft palate, and the floor of the mouth
- The *submental nodes* drain the lymphatics of the chin, part of the lower lip, the floor of the mouth, and the tip of the tongue

The nodal members of the pericervical collar drain essentially into the internal jugular chain; only the occipital lymph nodes drain into the spinal accessory chain.

1.3.5.2 Deep Cervical Nodes

For Rouvière (1932) the deep cervical lymph nodes include three different chains:

- The *internal jugular chain* is subdivided into anterior and lateral groups. The anterior nodes lie in front of the internal jugular vein, predominantly in the upper neck between the digastric muscle and the omohyoid muscle. Three divisions can be distinguished: a superior subdigastric group, often limited to a single large node (principal node of Küttner), which is the most frequent relay of upper aerodigestive tract cancers, a middle division (midjugular nodes) lying anterior to the thyrolinguofacial venous trunk, and an inferior division (low jugular nodes) located in the supraomohyoid region. The lateral group consists of smaller nodes; the uppermost members lie on the lateral aspect of the internal jugular vein while the lower nodes are found on the medial aspect. The internal jugular vein receives lymph either directly from the tissues or indirectly, after passage through outlying nodes, from the nasal fossa, tonsils, tongue, hard palate, thyroid gland, ear, submandibular gland, and sublingual glands.
- The *spinal accessory chain* consists of 8 to 10 nodes; it lies obliquely (superior to inferior, anterior to posterior) along the general course of the spinal accessory nerve, and is divided into two groups; the upper group blends with the superior internal jugular vein nodes while the lower group becomes continuous with the transverse cervical chain.
- The *transverse cervical chain* (supraclavicular chain) also follows an oblique course (lateral to medial); lying behind the clavicle, the transverse nodes prolong the lower end of the spinal accessory chain up to the thoracic duct on the left and the lymphatic duct on the right. This chain comprises 8–10 nodes; the most medial on the left is related to the subdiaphragmatic lymph pathways by the thoracic duct.

1.3.5.3 Accessory Chain Nodes

The accessory chains include both superficial chains and deep juxtavisceral chains:

- the *superficial chains* are satellites of the anterior jugular vein and the external jugular vein
- the *deep juxtavisceral chains* are inaccessible to both physical examination and ultrasonography. They include the lateral retropharyngeal nodes, one or two prelaryngeal (cricothyroid) nodes, the pretracheal nodes, and and the nodes of the recurrent chain.

1.3.5.4 Reporting Sonographic Data

In agreement with the surgeon and the histopathologist, it is practical to divide the lateral neck into eight different zones. As it is easier to localize the neck vessels, and particularly the carotid bifurcation, than the cervical muscles, nodes anterior to the major neurovascular bundle (common carotid artery, deep jugular vein, vagus nerve) can be termed jugular nodes, while nodes lying behind this bundle can be considered spinal nodes. Using height in the neck as a criterion, nodes situated at the level of the carotid bifurcation or above can be termed superior nodes, those lying 3 cm below the carotid bifurcation can be considered middle jugular or spinal nodes, and those located between the clavicle and the middle region can be referred to as inferior nodes. Along with a written report on sonographic findings, the sonographer should indicate the exact site and maximum diameter of any abnormal nodes detected by US on a surgical map. In addition to being an asset for the surgeon, such maps constitute a helpful reference document for the sonographer in the follow-up of nodal masses treated nonsurgically (Fig. 1.21).

1.4 References

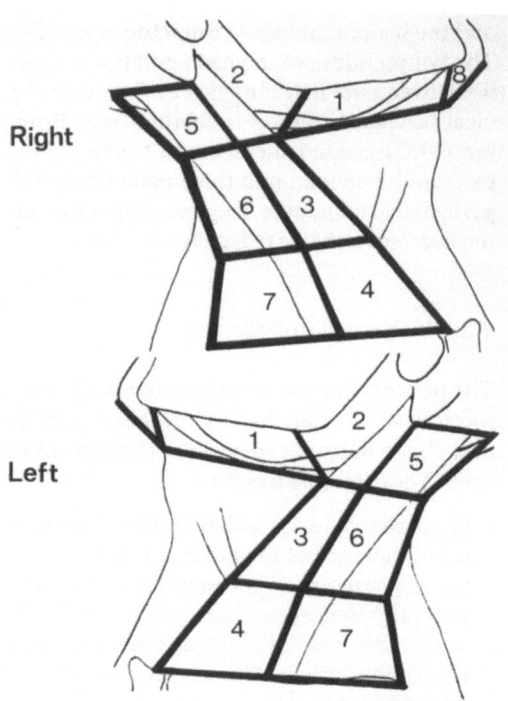

Fig. 1.21. Map for the follow-up of nodal masses treated nonsurgically

Bismuth V, Fendler JP, Grellet J, Blery M, Gaux JC (1975) Le diagnostic artériographique des adénomes parathyroïdiens. A propos de 45 cas. J Radiol 56: 235–244

Bruneton JN, Roux P, Caramella E, Demard F, Vallicioni J, Chauvel P (1984) Ear, nose and throat cancer: ultrasound diagnosis of metastasis to cervical lymph nodes. Radiology 152: 771–773

Bruneton JN, Roux P, Caramella E, Manzino JJ, Vallicioni J, Demard F (1986) Tongue and tonsil cancer: staging with US. Radiology 158: 743–746

Castleman B, Roth SI (1978) Tumors of the parathyroid glands. Atlas of tumor pathology, 2nd series, Fasc 14. AFIP Ed, Washington DC, pp 3–20

Hegedus L, Parrild H, Poulsen L, Andersen J, Holm B (1982) The determination of thyroid volume by ultrasound and its relationship to body weight, age and sex in normal subjects. J Clin Endocrinol Metab 56: 260–263

Leopold GR (1980) Ultrasonography of superficially located structures. Radiol Clin North Am 18: 161–173

McGahan JP, Walter JP (1985) Aspiration-biopsy procedure: comparison of ultrasound guidance methods. J Ultrasound Med 4: 158

Moreau JF, Carlier-Conrads L (1984) Imagerie diagnostique des glandes thyroíde et parathyroides. Vigot, Paris, pp 33–40

Benson DM, Rifkin MD, Rose JL, Goldberg BB (1983) Characterization of benign and malignant tissues of the thyroid gland. An ultrasonic approach using RF waveform analysis and pattern recognition. Invest Radiol 18: 459–462

Poncin-Viateau J, Hassan M (1985) Echographie thyroïdienne. Vigot, Paris, pp 33–45

Rizzatto G, Solbiati L, Derchi LE (1985) The use of a biopsy intraoperative probe to guide fine needle biopsy of superficially located lesions. J Ultrasound Med 4: 177

Rouvière H (1932) Anatomie des lymphatiques de l'homme. Masson, Paris

Sample WF, Mitchell SP, Bledsoe RC (1979) Parathyroid ultrasonography. Radiology 127: 485–490

Shawker TH, Sonies B, Stone M, Garra B (1985) Ultrasound examination of speech and swallowing. J Ultrasound Med 4: 155

Tannahil A, Hooper M, England M, Ferris J, Wilson M (1978) Measurement of thyroid size by ultrasound, palpation and scintiscan. Clin Endocrinol 8: 483–486

Wang CA (1976) The anatomic basis of parathyroid surgery. Ann Surg 183: 271–275

2 Thyroid Gland

J.-N. BRUNETON AND F. NORMAND

This chapter deals with congenital malformations and tumors of the thyroid gland, inflammatory pathologies, thyroid dysfunction, and the problems specific to the postsurgery thyroid.

2.1 Congenital Malformations

Aside from thyroid agenesis and ectopia in children (cf. Chap. 7), thyroid anomalies are basically limited to agenesis or hypoplasia of a lobe.

Lobe agenesis occurs in less than 0.1% of the population (Greening et al. 1980). The malformation is an incidental discovery during cervical examinations for another pathology or when the existing lobe is the site of an anomaly. On sonograms, the fat tissue which replaces the absent lobe is imaged as an area of dense, irregular echoes; the common carotid artery and the internal jugular vein lie near the trachea. Females are affected more often than males, and the left lobe is more apt to be missing than the right lobe. Apart from the possibility of an anomaly induced by the existing lobe, agenesis of a thyroid lobe has no functional implications.

Hypoplasia of a thyroid lobe is more frequent, and is easily recognized sonographically by the asymmetry of images on transverse scans (difference of at least 50% between the size of the two lobes) (fig. 2.1). This malformation has no impact on gland function either.

2.2 Thyroid Tumors and Goiter

In addition to a review of the general features of goiter and thyroid tumors and a discussion of the imaging techniques (including nonultrasonographic procedures) available for etiologi-

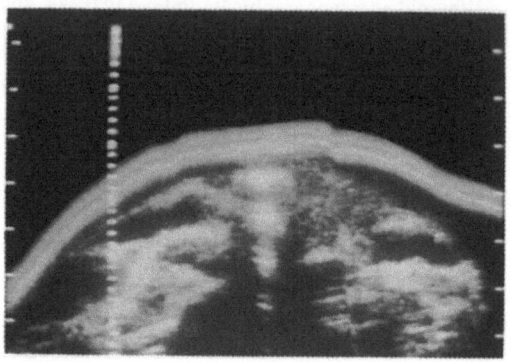

Fig. 2.1. Hypoplasia of the right thyroid lobe (transverse scan)

cal diagnosis, the sonographic characteristics of both benign and malignant processes are presented here. The exploratory protocol proposed is based on an awareness of the possibilities and limitations of thyroid sonography.

Ultrasonography is a highly sensitive technique for the detection of subclinical nodules. Owing to the prevalence of occult disease, the exploratory approach must be individualized for each patient, taking into account the medical history, clinical context, ultrasonographic (US) appearance, and any aspiration cytology findings (Bruneton and Caramella 1984).

2.2.1 General Features

2.2.1.1 Diagnosis

More and more frequently, thyroid tumors are diagnosed before there are any clinical manifestations. This is particularly true for lesions found during examination of the cervical nodes as part of lymphoma workups or searches for a primary tumor. Discovery of one or more thyroid nodules during US and Doppler ultrasound examinations of the carotid artery is even more common (Carroll 1982).

Diffuse goiter refers to global enlargement of the thyroid gland as a result of thyroid dysfunction, which may or may not be symmetrical. The prospective clinical diagnosis depends on the nature of the gland enlargement. Physical examination and ultrasonography are used for evaluation. In homogeneous goiter the gland is more or less uniformly enlarged, despite a certain tendency towards asymmetry. On palpation, the gland has a smooth or slightly bosselated surface and a uniformly firm, rubbery consistency. Auscultation may demonstrate a vascular murmur. The presence or absence of any other associated signs, and in particular thyrotoxicosis, allows diagnosis by means of appropriately oriented tests.

Simple (nontoxic) goiter is a benign diffuse or multinodular thyroid enlargement without any apparent signs of gland dysfunction. Physical and biochemical tests usually confirm euthyroidism. Goiters resulting from deficient iodine intake (endemic goiter), excessive intake of goitrogens, or iatrogenic factors are rarely encountered today. A congenital iodide-trapping defect is another rare cause. Simple goiter affects females more often than males, and the typical patient is a young, neurodystonic woman who has been under physical stress or is in a period in which sex hormones play a major role (puberty, menopause, pregnancy, lactation).

The course of simple goiter is extremely variable; spontaneous regression is possible, but transformation into a chronic condition is more frequent. Chronic goiter may be complicated by endocrine disorders (thyrotoxicosis), tracheal compression (leading to progressive dyspnea), and, exceptionally, a vascular syndrome that should prompt a search for mediastinal thyroid tissue ("diving goiter"). Transformation of a goiter itself is actually more common, and intrathyroidal hemorrrhage or cystic degeneration (frequently massive) can be responsible for a pseudotumoral appearance. Less often, an inflammatory episode causes strumitis with an acute clinical picture (cf. Sect. 2.3). The major risk with simple goiter is malignant change, which should be suspected whenever rapid growth is noted.

There are also several other forms of goiter associated with hyperthyroidism, a fact which distinguishes them from Graves' disease, which affects a normal thyroid gland. These forms are noteworthy especially because of their clinical course. Cancer rarely occurs concomitantly with hyperthyroidism (less than 1% of all cases), but when such associations do exist the malignancy is apt to be an anaplastic carcinoma with a rapid course and a poor prognosis.

In *multinodular goiter*, the gland is diffusely enlarged; palpation detects a mass of variable consistency that can attain considerable dimensions; the gland surface is bosselated. The frequency of these gross features is at least partly explained by the fact that all diffuse goiters tend to become multinodular with time. Although these features classically suggest a benign lesion, the risk of malignant change is greater than for homogeneous goiters. Multinodular goiter can occur in three different clinical forms: colloid, toxic multinodular, and diffuse neoplastic goiter.

Colloid goiter is a form of simple goiter without any abnormal hormone secretion; lesions typically feel hard, whereas the rest of the thyroid tissue feels soft or fluctuant.

The isthmus is the site of predilection. Diagnosis may be suggested by endemic factors or the occasional context of goitrous cretinism. The disease course is similar to that of homogeneous goiter but there is a greater risk of compression-related complications because colloid goiters can reach substantial size. Hemorrhage is another major problem. Other possible complications include strumitis, progression to toxicosis, and malignant change.

Toxic multinodular goiter is associated with thyrotoxicosis. The markedly enlarged gland contains both toxic nodules and nonfunctioning zones. This pathology essentially affects women over 50 years of age, and develops in a healthy gland or a euthyroid multinodular goiter during a period of stress or intense sex hormone activity (puberty, menopause, pregnancy, etc.).

Diffuse neoplastic goiter corresponds to an advanced form of thyroid cancer (usually a poorly differentiated type). Diagnosis is made clinically. Tumors vary in size but are usually quite large. Tumoral involvement may predominate in a nontender or slightly inflammatory lobe with a hard consistency and an inhomogeneous, bosselated surface. Whereas older patients may report a long-standing history of goiter, any rapid change is cause for alarm. On physical examination, thyroid mobility is restricted when the patient swallows. Advanced lesions may more or less completely enclose peritumoral nodes. Rapid growth of a goiter can cause dysphonia (owing to damage to the recurrent laryngeal nerve), progressive dyspnea, and occasionally even dysphagia. The diagnosis is clinically patent, and the major concern is deciding whether or not the patient is a good candidate for surgery.

Nodular tumors of the thyroid gland cause the most difficulties in diagnosis. The nodule may manifest as a focal, well-circumscribed, clinically palpable swelling or merely tumefaction of an otherwise normal gland. Nodular tumors are generally discovered fortuitously and are quite common; the estimated incidence in the United States is 6%. Both long-standing and recent nodules can be differentiated from enlarged lymph nodes by the fact that they move along with the larynx when the patient swallows. Nodular tumors tend to have a firm, rubbery consistency; hard masses are seen occasionally, but soft tumors are exceptional. Most nodular tumors occur in a thyroid lobe; isthmic lesions are less common. Regardless of the site, these tumors are nontender.

Along with the patient's age and sex, the history should include his or her geographic origin and any relevant personal or familial antecedents. Particular note must be made of any previous relevant treatments such as cervical irradiation during childhood. The date of discovery of the nodule, its growth pattern (gradual or rapid), and any associated local regional signs (pain, dyspnea, dysphonia, dysphagia) are other important factors for diagnosis. Local examination, including visual evaluation and palpation, assesses the location, size, consistency, and mobility of the nodule. All of the cervical node regions must be explored to detect any nodal involvement.

Based on the topographic data provided by US, and the functional information obtained by radionuclide scanning, lesions can be classed as a "hot" nodule, with the clinical picture of toxic adenoma, a "hot" nontoxic nodule or solitary nodule, or a "cold" nodule. This last type involves the most problems for the clinician. Whether accompanied or not by hyperthyroidism, "hot" nodules are only rarely associated with a neoplastic process (less than 1% of cases); by contrast, "cold" nodules have a much higher incidence of malignancy (10%–20% of cases). Aside from cancerous lesions, the most frequent etiology is a benign adenoma.

The various clinical pictures described above are those encountered by the clinician; the sonographer should be familiar with them so that he can efficiently orient the etiological search (Mazzaferri 1981).

2.2.1.2 Pathologic Classification

In addition to epithelial and nonepithelial tumors, various secondary and pseudotumoral lesions affect the thyroid gland. The majority of benign epithelial tumors are follicular adenomas; embryonal, fetal, simple, colloid, oxyphilic, and atypical epithelial tumors are less frequent. Malignant epithelial thyroid tumors include follicular carcinoma, papillary carcinoma, undifferentiated (anaplastic) carcinoma, and medullary carcinoma. Both benign and malignant nonepithelial tumors are rare. Fibrosarcomas account for most malignancies; the other thyroid neoplasms include carcinosarcoma, malignant hemangioendothelioma, lymphoma, and teratoma. Metastasis to the thyroid gland is rare. Pseudotumoral lesions include a variety of pathological entities: ectopic thyroid tissue, intrathyroid cysts, adenomatous goiter, Graves' disease, thyroiditis, amyloid goiter, and squamous metaplasia. A constellation of clinical and biological findings generally suffices for diagnosis.

2.2.1.3 TNM Classification

The TNM system for tumor classification is based on both clinical and sonographic data (Gerard-Marchand 1977).

T - Primary Tumor

T0   no visible or palpable tumor
T1   single nodule in one lobe with or without gland deformity and with no limitation of mobility; T1s single nodule; T1m multiple nodules
T2   bilateral tumor with or without deformity of the gland and with no limitation of mobility; T2s single nodule of the isthmus
T3   unilateral, bilateral, or isthmic tumor with extension beyond the gland capsule and invasion of adjacent structures

The data obtained from nodal explorations allows classification as follows:

N - Regional Lymph Nodes

N0   no palpable node
N1   movable homolateral lymph node; N1a node not suspicious for malignancy; N1b node suspicious for malignancy
N2   movable contralateral, midline, or bilateral node; N2a nodes not suspicious for malignancy; N2b nodes suspicious for malignancy
N3   fixed nodes

After a thorough disease workup, distant metastases are classified as follows:

M - Distant Metastases

M0   no evidence of distant metastasis
M1   evidence of distant metastasis

Ultrasonography is a more sensitive technique than physical examination for determination of T and N categories, and has had an impact on tumor staging. In the future, both the presentation of therapeutic results and classifications will probably include reference to ultrasound data, something that was unthought of in studies performed 5 or more years ago.

2.2.2 Nonultrasonographic Techniques of Thyroid Exploration

2.2.2.1 Thyroid Function Tests

For many years, thyroid function was evaluated using iodine-131, but the indications for this technique are now limited, owing to the introduction of circulating thyroid hormone assays and measurement of thyroid-stimulating hormone (TSH) levels.

All of the various hormones secreted by the thyroid can be quantified by radioimmunoassays, but only *thyroxine (T$_4$)* and *triiodothyronine (T$_3$)* levels are of diagnostic value for determination of euthyroidism, hyperthyroidism, or hypothyroidism. The normal range for T$_4$ is 65-140 nmol/liter, and that for T$_3$ is 1-3 nmol/liter. T$_3$ transport can be assessed by assaying thyroxine-binding globulin (TBG) levels, and by determining the free T$_4$ index and free hormone concentrations.

Thyroglobulin levels are determined by radioimmunoassay in the absence of antithyroglobulin antibodies (Pacini et al. 1980). In normal individuals, the thyroglobulin concentration varies from 5-30 ng/ml. Numerous pathologies are characterized by elevated thyroglobulin levels; this is particularly true of hyperthyroidism, whatever its origin. The thyroglobulin level of "cold" nodules lacks histopathological specificity, i.e., it cannot distinguish adenoma from cancer. By contrast, thyroglobulin assays are essential for the follow-up of patients with differentiated thyroid cancers: serum thyroglobulin should be undetectable in patients whose thyroid has been completely destroyed, and thus its presence is indicative of malignant tissue. Stimulation by TSH increases the sensitivity of thyroglobulin tests. In patients with residual normal thyroid tissue, an elevation in the thyroglobulin level during suppressive treatment suggests metastasis (Schlumberger et al. 1981).

Exploration of the *hypothalamic-pituitary axis* is based on measurement of the TSH level (normal range 1-10 μU/ml) and the thyrotrophin-releasing hormone (TRH) test. The TRH test is indicated when hyperthyroidism is suspected.

Radioactive iodine uptake tests are useful for the workup of hyperthyroid patients when radioiodine treatment is envisaged.

The other most important thyroid test is determination of *antithyroid antibody titers;* antithyroglobulin antibodies and antimicrosomial antibodies are the two substances most frequently assayed on a routine basis for patients with thyroiditis. Investigations for patients with Graves' disease include measurement of *long-acting thyroid stimulator (LATS) immunoglobulins.*

2.2.2.2 Non-US, Non-CT Imaging Techniques

Radionuclide scanning of the thyroid gland currently makes use of three different radioelements:

- iodine-131 is a relatively inexpensive scanning agent, but delivers a high radiation dose for a scintiscan; its use is therefore restricted to studies prior to treatment with iodine-131 and the follow-up of differentiated thyroid cancers
- iodine-123 is only employed on a limited basis for thyroid scans as production of this radionuclide is hampered by problems with contamination and its high cost
- ^{99}Tc-pertechnetate is trapped by the thyroid but is not organified. Satisfactory scans can be obtained 20 min after intravenous product injection. ^{99}Tc-pertechnetate is the most commonly used radionuclide for thyroid studies owing to its dosimetric advantages (short half-life) and ease of use.

Scintigraphy is useful for tumoral investigations as it can assess the functional status of a thyroid nodule (nonfunctioning or autonomous). Technetium advantageously solves the major problems of scintigraphy (cost, radiation dose) in most cases. When technetium scans are insufficiently contrasted, use of iodine-123 is advisable; this is the case for mediastinal thyroids, mediastinal masses (although CT is probably better for such cases), and ectopic (especially lingual) thyroids. Iodine-131 is fundamental for the follow-up of patients with a differentiated thyroid cancer; scans are obtained 72 h after product administration. Slow scanning of the cervical region and then of the whole body using a multitransducer scintigraphy unit allows evaluation of any product concentration by thyroid metastases.

Fluorescent thyroid imaging is an alternative exploratory procedure that can be used for patients with iodine saturation and for pregnant women.

Transverse axial tomoscintigraphy promises to become a highly accurate diagnostic procedure in the future, in particular when combined with use of labelled monoclonal antibodies raised against the carcinoembryonic antigen (CEA), for example, for the localization of medullary cancer.

Soft ray cervical radiography can demonstrate fine calcifications in cases of thyroid cancer, and especially papillary types. Larger, less uniform calcifications can be detected in cases of adenoma, and particularly in long-standing lesions. *Chest X-rays* are a valuable means of evaluating the mediastinal nature of a goiter as well as its impact on the direction and caliber of the trachea.

2.2.2.3 Computed Tomography

While the indications for ultrasonography are constantly increasing due to the technique's excellent sensitivity for the detection of small lesions, CT is basically limited to the workup of thyroid cancers, diagnosis of mediastinal thyroid tissue, and in vivo determination of the iodine content. Although thyroid cancer may be clinically patent, CT is useful for detecting metastatic cervical nodes, and whether or not they thrombose the internal jugular vein (although

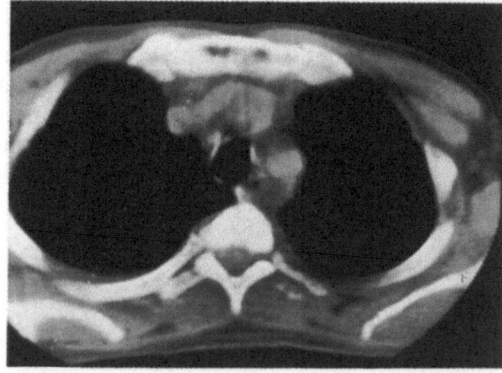

Fig. 2.2. CT scan of metastatic nodes in the anterior superior mediastinum *(dotted lines)* in a patient with thyroid cancer

diagnosis is easier and faster with US). CT is especially useful for localizing nodal masses in the anterior superior mediastinum (Fig. 2.2) and evaluating thyroid relations with the trachea. CT exploration of the mediastinum is also indicated for the detection of nodal involvement after intraoperative discovery of thyroid cancer. CT is warranted during the follow-up of patients with thyroid cancer if there are signs suggestive of local disease recurrence, as malignancy can spread to the trachea, mediastinum, or sternum (Radecki et al. 1984).

"Diving" goiters, representing mediastinal thyroid tissue, are associated with a mediastinal syndrome; the anterior mediastinum is affected more often than the posterior mediastinum. Scintiscans are not always positive for these sites, whereas CT is rarely unsuccessful. For Glazer et al. (1982) the CT characteristics of mediastinal thyroid tissue include anatomic continuity with the cervical thyroid, a CT number greater than 100 HU, occasionally with focal calcifications, pronounced enhancement greater than that of lymph nodes after injection of contrast material, and prolonged enhancement (longer than 2 min). Data obtained by CT for this pathology often obviates the need for exploratory thoracotomy.

The average density (CT number) of the thyroid is related to the gland's iodine content, and varies as a function of the exogenous iodine supply and the gland's iodide trapping capacity. The iodine concentration can be determined by analysis of gland density on CT scans.

The value of CT for thyroid pathologies is currently dominated by two indications: pre- and postoperative evaluation of thyroid cancers, and the diagnosis and workup of mediastinal thyroids (Silverman et al. 1984).

2.2.2.4 Aspiration Cytology

The frequency of use of aspiration cytology for thyroid tumors varies from one country to another. The largest series can probably be credited to Sweden, where this technique has been common practice for over 30 years. Cytologic puncture must be both atraumatic and produce material sufficiently rich in cells to allow satisfactory interpretation. Although certain teams advocate use of large calibre needles, fine-nee-

dle aspiration seems sufficient when performed correctly. Neither local anesthesia nor cutaneous incision are required; the skin is simply prepared with an antiseptic solution, and puncture performed after cutaneous or ultrasonographic localization. Various aspiration techniques have been advocated: a fine needle mounted on a syringe, blockable piston syringe, etc. Other authors simply use a needle, which is withdrawn as soon as a drop of fluid rises in the tip.

Cytologic examination of thyroid aspirate smears takes several factors into account: cellular morphology, size and appearance of cell clumps, differences in the size of cells and nuclei, extent of any cell anomalies, and the nature of adjacent elements (macrophages, lymphocytes, connective tissue). The difficulties encountered in cytological interpretation of thyroid biopsies can be briefly summarized as follows:

- adenoma and well-differentiated follicular carcinoma: when well-differentiated thyroid cells are present, the problem is their identification because they are sometimes morphologically similar to the cells of benign adenoma
- moderately differentiated follicular carcinoma and papillary carcinoma generally involve fewer diagnostic problems (Miller et al. 1981)
- undifferentiated carcinomas are usually easy to diagnose by cytology
- undifferentiated small cell carcinoma and malignant lymphoma: although the malignant nature of the lesion leaves no doubt, the differential diagnosis can be difficult
- thyroiditis and carcinoma: the morphological modifications that occur in thyroid cells during Hashimoto's disease can be mistaken for carcinoma
- lymphoma and Hashimoto's thyroiditis: the extensive immunoblastic hyperplasia observed in Hashimoto's disease may be misinterpreted as malignant lymphoma

Fine needle aspiration biopsy is sufficiently reliable for clinicians to select medical surveillance or surgery on the basis of the cytology report. Only some 15% of biopsies fail to produce enough cellular material for proper examination; cytology findings for the 85% of successful biopsies concur with histology 81%–92% of the time (Block et al. 1983; Heim et al. 1984; Jennings and Atkinson 1983; Lo Gerfo et al. 1982; Prinz et al. 1983). False negative errors of malignancy generally correspond to well-differentiated follicular carcinomas that have been misdiagnosed as adenomas.

Cytological puncture after cutaneous localization has been successfully employed throughout the world; owing to the increasing frequency at which asymptomatic thyroid nodules are now being detected, ultrasonic localization seems advisable.

2.2.3 Ultrasonography

Because high frequency US can detect fluid-filled nodules as small as 1 mm in diameter and solid, hypoechogenic nodules of at least 2–3 mm, it is much more sensitive than either physical examination or scintigraphy. However, while it can demonstrate the gross features of tumors, it cannot differentiate the histologic types; the semiological characteristics of thyroid nodules must be analyzed (Cole-Beuglet and Goldberg 1983; Katz et al. 1984; Leopold 1980; Moreau and Carlier-Conrads 1984; Scheible et al. 1979; Simeone et al. 1982; Solbiati et al. 1985; Stark et al. 1983).

2.2.3.1 US Pattern

A lesion's sonographic pattern depends on its internal structure:

- *pure cysts* manifest sonographically as anechogenic structures with considerable posterior reinforcement. Cyst walls are usually thin, and no solid component is visible, even when the gain setting is increased (Fig. 2.3). This last point is important, as a lesion that contains some solid tissue may appear anechogenic if the gain is too low, either because the cyst fluid is thick or because the cyst contains hemorrhagic material.
- evaluation of *solid, homogeneous nodules* relies on comparison with the adjacent healthy parenchyma for definition of hyper-, iso-, or hypoechogenicity (Figs. 2.4–2.6). Hypoechogenic nodules predominate statistically.

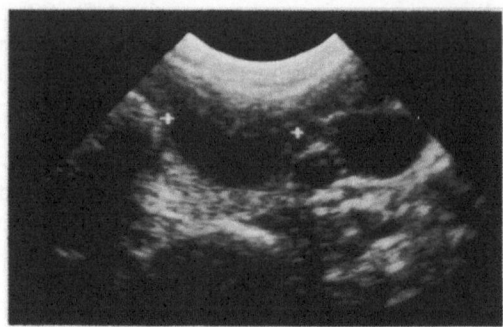

Fig. 2.3. Anechogenic thyroid cysts with posterior reinforcement (transverse scan of the left thyroid lobe; the common carotid artery and the internal jugular vein are seen in transverse section, lateral to the thyroid cyst)

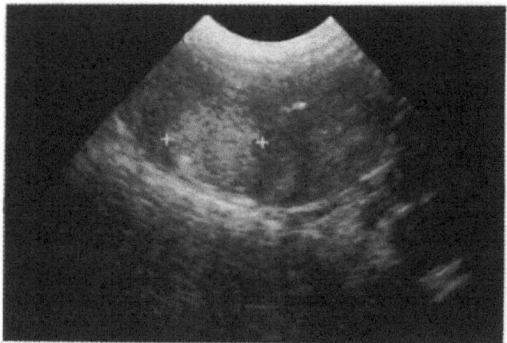

Fig. 2.4. Hyperechogenic nodule

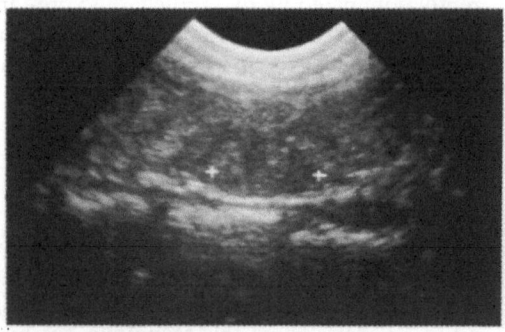

Fig. 2.5. Isoechogenic nodule (15 mm between the two *crosses*)

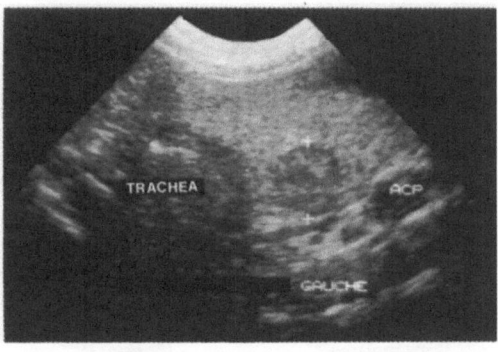

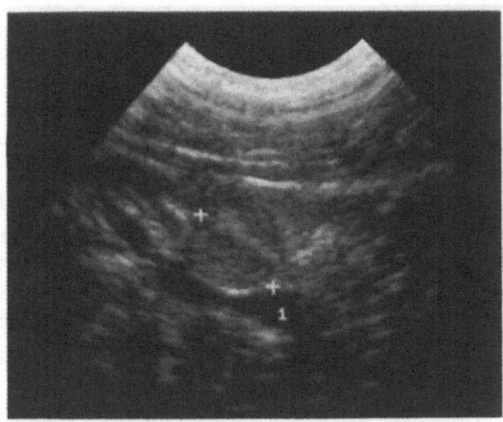

 Fig. 2.6. Hypoechogenic nodule (12 mm between the two *crosses*) on a transverse scan of the left thyroid lobe. *ACP,* common carotid artery

 Fig. 2.8. Thyroid nodule bounded laterally by the superior thyroid artery *(1)* and medially by a halo (11 mm between the two *crosses*)

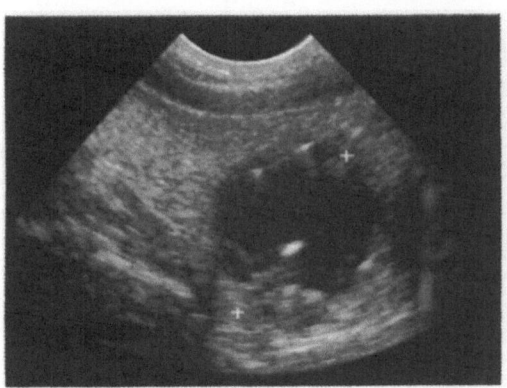

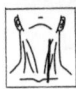 **Fig. 2.7.** Solid lesion that has undergone hemorrhagic involution (29 mm between the two *crosses*)

dule in which the fluid component predominates; these essentially fluid-filled nodules can be distinguished from true cysts by their solid wall. They may contain septa or even parietal protuberances, which must not be confused with malignant change in a cyst. Comparison of wall dimensions with the overall size of the lesion allows definition of the wall/nodule ratio; ratios under 25% usually correspond to necrotic adenomas.
- *calcifications* have a variety of sonographic appearances; calcifications smaller than 100 μ are visualized as small, echogenic punctate images on the periphery or inside a nodule. Macrocalcifications are always readily imaged as strongly echogenic forms with a sharply marginated acoustic shadow.

Solid, homogeneous nodules may show posterior attenuation, absence of posterior reinforcement, or posterior reinforcement (this last sign is thus not specific to anechogenic nodules).
- *"mixed" nodules* are often actually solid lesions that have undergone cystic or hemorrhagic degeneration (Fig. 2.7), and the respective percentages of the solid and fluid components must be determined. The term "false cyst" has been used by Poncin-Viateau and Hassan (1985) to designate a mixed no-

2.2.3.2 Nodule Margins

In addition to their internal structure, nodules are characterized by the nature (sharply or ill defined) of their margins. A peripheral halo of decreased echogenicity may be present, especially around iso- and hyperechogenic nodules. These halos correspond to a thin hypoechogenic rim separating the tumor from healthy tissue. Although this halo sign is not pathognomonic for benignity, it is a reasonably good indicator of a nonneoplastic process (Fig. 2.8).

2.2.3.3 Ultrasonographic Consistency of Nodules

On physical examination nodules can be classified as soft, fluctuant, or hard; the clinical appraisal can be verified visually from sonograms. Deformation of the tumor or normal peripheral thyroid tissue can be detected by pressing the transducer down against the skin over the site of the lesion. Compressible tumors tend to be adenomatous rather than malignant; this is particularly true for solid lesions.

2.2.3.4 Number of Nodules

The sensitivity of thorough thyroid sonography covering both lobes and the isthmus is unequalled by any other preoperative technique for the localization of nodules. In our experience (Bruneton et al. 1985), ultrasound is nearly as sensitive as intraoperative palpation. Although the therapeutic protocol may depend on whether lesions appear uni- or multifocal, this information is particularly useful in orienting the operative procedure when surgery is indicated. Well-circumscribed nodules can easily be counted by US and localized with respect to healthy tissue. In adenomatous goiter, however, it is hard to sonographically demonstrate normal tissue among more or less large nodular formations with variable US patterns.

2.2.3.5 Localization of Nodules

Determination of the exact location of a solitary nodule is less important than localization of diffuse lesions. Indeed, when surgery is indicated, the surgeon must know whether the superior poles of the thyroid lobes are intact, as this is a prerequisite for subtotal thyroidectomy. Indication of US-determined nodule locations and thyroid lobe dimensions on a diagram can be of considerable assistance for therapeutic decisions, especially when not all lesions are palpable. Such diagrams are also valuable reference documents for sonographic follow-up of medically managed patients (Fig. 2.9).

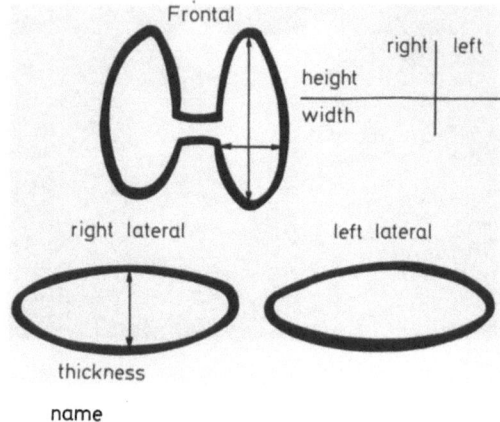

Fig. 2.9. Thyroid lobe dimensions. The locations, number, and diameters of nodules are indicated by the sonographer

2.2.3.6 Exploration of the Lateral Cervical Nodes

Ultrasonographic examination of the thyroid gland is not complete without a systematic search for enlarged jugulocarotid nodes. The presence of one or more enlarged nodes together with a thyroid nodule is a good indication of malignancy, especially since US evaluation of lymph nodes, like thyroid sonography, is more sensitive than physical examination (cf. Chap. 5).

2.2.4 Benign Tumors of the Thyroid Gland

Benign tumors of the thyroid include adenomas and cysts. True thyroid cysts are quite rare, and most so-called cystic lesions are actually completely necrotic or cystic adenomas.

2.2.4.1 Adenoma (Figs. 2.10–2.22)

Almost all benign thyroid tumors are adenomas, which arise from follicular epithelium and can be divided into follicular (the most frequent) and papillary types. These well-encapsulated tumors lie within and displace the normal parenchyma. Adenomas may be either solitary or multiple (as in adenomatous goiter).

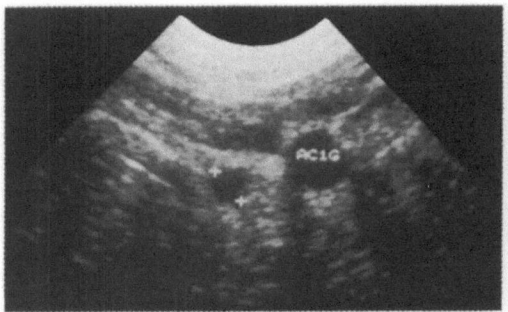

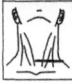

Fig.2.10. Small hypoechogenic adenoma of the left thyroid lobe (transverse scan). *ACIG*, left common carotid artery

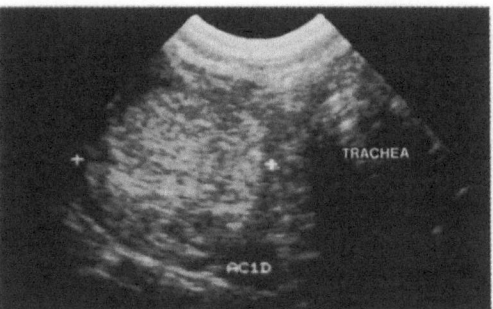

Fig.2.12. Large hyperechogenic nodule of the right thyroid lobe displacing the right carotid artery *(ACID)* posteriorly (31 mm between the two *crosses*)

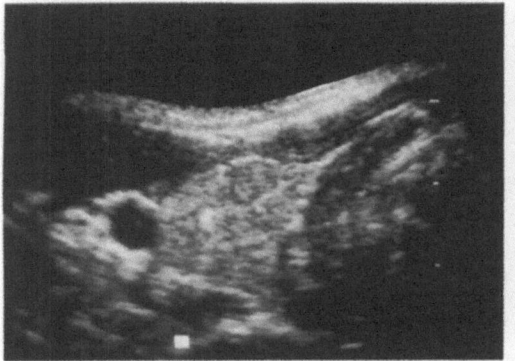

Fig.2.11. Small isoechogenic adenoma recognizable solely by the peripheral halo (transverse scan of the right lobe)

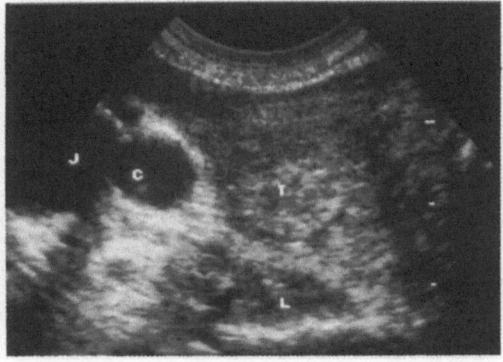

Fig.2.13. Hyperechogenic nodule of the left thyroid lobe (transverse scan). *C*, primary carotid artery; *J*, internal jugular vein; *L*, longus colli muscle; *T*, adenoma

Hyperfunctioning "toxic" adenomas are characterized by predominantly cellular hyperplasia. Abundant colloid deposits, on the other hand, can result in capsular breakthrough and the formation of thyroid cysts. One-third of all adenomas explored by US show some degree of cystic or necrotic degeneration. Adenomatous calcifications, when present, are usually thick and irregular.

The diversity of the sonographic patterns encountered for adenomas reflects the multiplicity of anatomic forms and the variability in the number of lesions. Adenomatous nodules can be classified as hypo-, iso-, or hyperechogenic. An isoechogenic nodule may escape US detection even if it is clinically palpable; the repeat examination required in such cases using a water bath or Reston interface can demonstrate superficial lesions owing to the presence of a halo or a discrete difference in echogenicity relative to the healthy thyroid tissue. Along with these different patterns, cystic degeneration, necrosis, and hemorrhagic processes are visualized as more or less irregular, anechogenic images, and occasionally as solid nodules with internal septations. The amount of fluid in adenomas varies considerably; the fluid component may represent only a small percentage of the entire mass or the lesion may be entirely cystic. Intratumoral hemorrhage responsible for pain of sudden onset or rapid growth of a known nodule is suggested when sonograms depict an anechogenic zone which is considerably larger than the nodule's solid component.

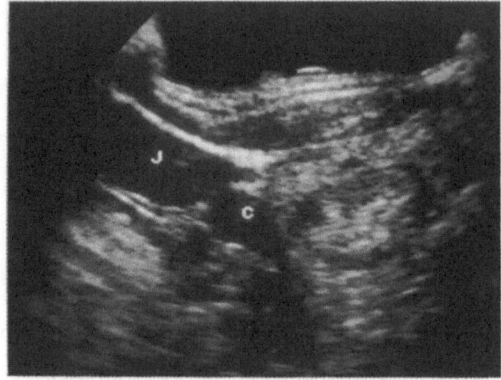

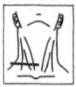 **Fig. 2.14.** Halo sign in thyroid adenoma. *C,* common carotid artery; *J,* internal jugular vein

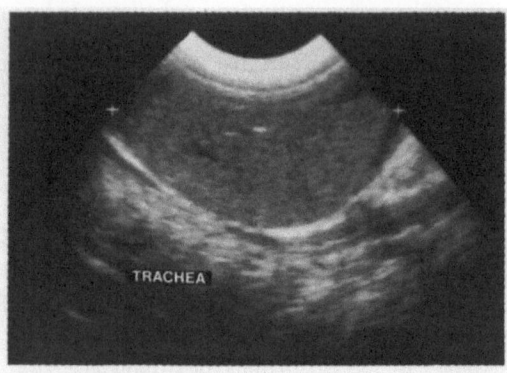

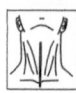 **Fig. 2.17.** Adenoma of the pyramidal lobe (sagittal scan of the midportion of the neck, anterior to the trachea) (45 mm between the two crosses)

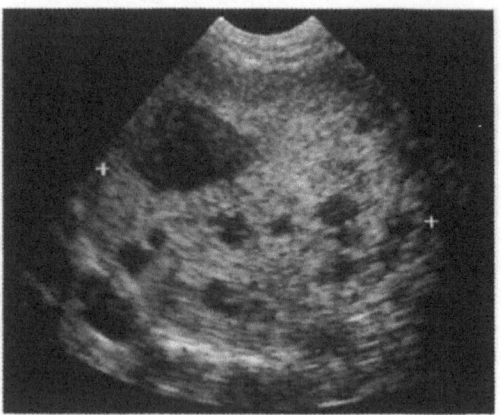

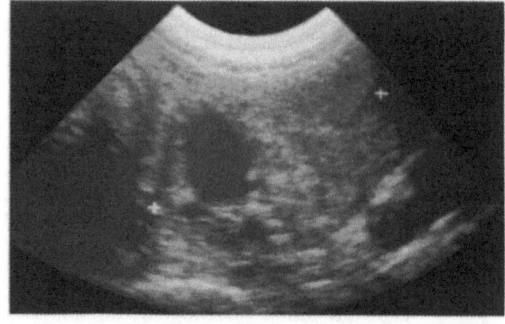

 Fig. 2.18. Partially necrotic adenoma (transverse scan) (34 mm between the two *crosses*)

 Fig. 2.15. Large adenoma with multiple necrotic zones (74 mm between the two *crosses*)

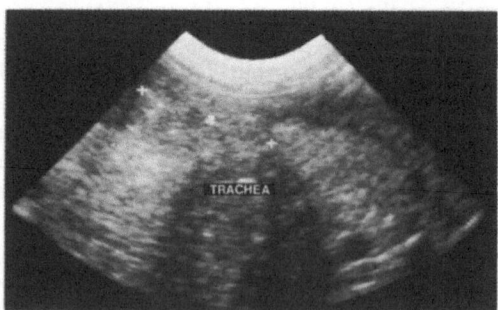

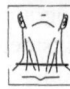 **Fig. 2.16.** Adenoma on the right of the isthmus (transverse scan) (21 mm between the two *crosses*)

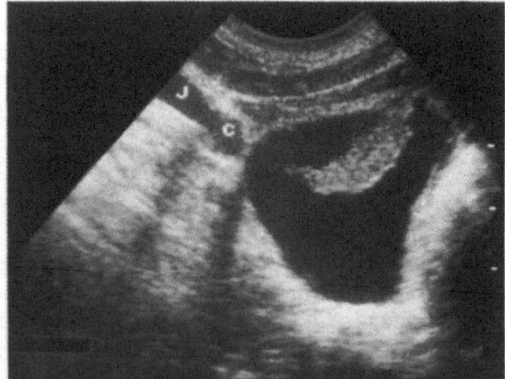

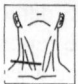 **Fig. 2.19.** Necrotic adenoma. *C,* common carotid artery; *J,* internal jugular vein

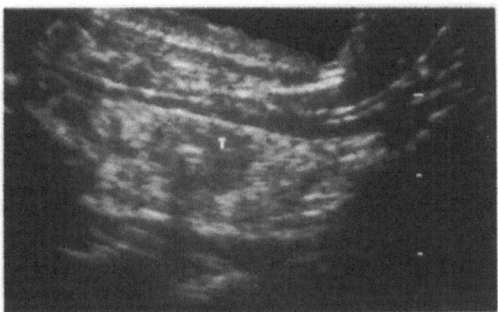

Fig. 2.22. Small central calcification (echogenic image with an acoustic shadow) in an adenoma (sagittal scan of the left thyroid lobe)

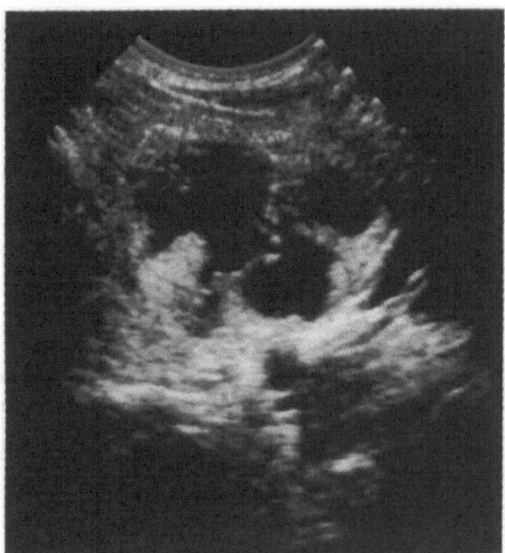

Fig. 2.20. Necrotic adenoma

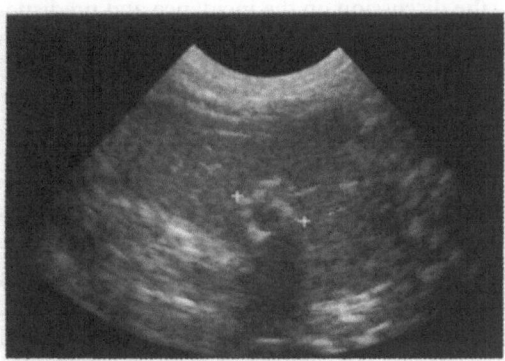

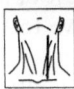
Fig. 2.21. Calcified adenoma

Adenomatous calcifications are readily demonstrated on sonograms as strongly echogenic images with sharp margins and an acoustic shadow; calcifications are most apt to occur in known lesions, and especially in adenomatous goiter. The sonographic pattern of adenomatous goiter can be extremely complex. The major interest of ultrasound is evaluation of thyroid volume and the search for any sonographically homogeneous zones corresponding to

healthy tissue rather than determination of the exact number and pattern of lesions.

Whether palpable or not, scintigraphically "cold" nodules can be managed medically, as administration of a sufficiently high dose of thyroid hormone suppresses the effect of endogenous TSH. Three-month treatment courses can produce regression of nearly 50% in lesion size and even complete nodule disappearance for certain TSH-dependent adenomas, namely those that appear sonographically solid. By contrast, no modifications can be expected in the size of nodules with a cystic or hemorrhagic component; such cases require analysis by fine needle aspiration biopsy if surgery is not performed immediately.

2.2.4.2 Thyroid Cysts (Fig. 2.23–2.25)

Excluding cases of complete cystic degeneration of an adenoma, true thyroid cysts are rare. On sonograms these well-defined anechogenic masses exhibit posterior reinforcement. Hemorrhage into a cyst can be the origin of small echoes which complicate sonographic interpretation.

The frequency of carcinomatous change in small cystic lesions is only around 2% (Allen et al. 1979; Beckers 1979). Cysts smaller than 4 cm in greatest dimension and lesions without internal septations or intracystic growths are amenable to aspiration biopsy. For all other "cystic" lesions, including cysts that have reformed af-

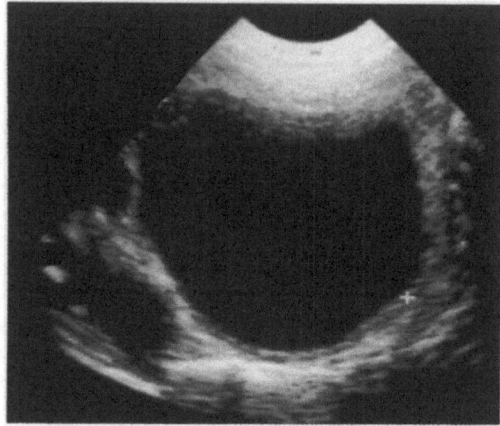

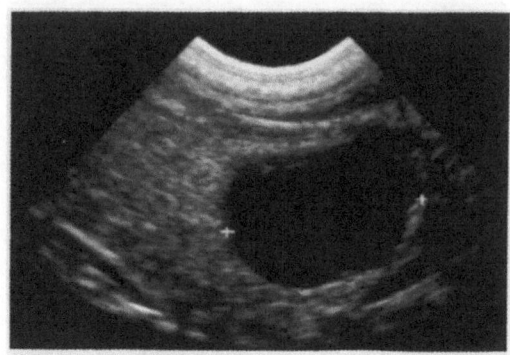

Fig. 2.23. Thyroid cyst

Fig. 2.25. Complete cystic degeneration of an adenoma. This anechogenic structure closely resembles a cyst; histological examination was required to obtain the correct etiology

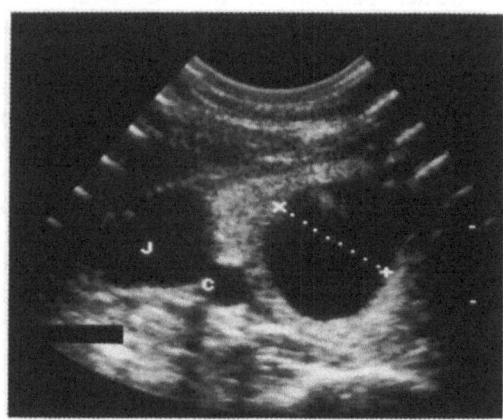

Fig. 2.24. Thyroid cyst (transverse scan). *C*, common carotid artery; *J*, internal jugular vein

ter an initial puncture, surgical excision remains the procedure of choice.

2.2.5 Malignant Tumors of the Thyroid Gland

In addition to reviewing the etiological characteristics and predisposing factors of thyroid cancer, this section describes well-differentiated follicular adenocarcinoma, moderately differentiated follicular adenocarcinoma, ana-

plastic carcinoma, medullary carcinoma, metastases, lymphomas, and sarcomas. These last three etiologies are rare, and the greater part of the discussion on the incidence and predisposing factors of thyroid malignancies concerns follicular and undifferentiated carcinomas.

2.2.5.1 Epidemiology and Etiology

The exact frequency of thyroid cancer is hard to determine because occult cancers are extremely common, as demonstrated by autopsy series. Vidone and Silverberg (1966) have estimated that thyroid malignancies represent only 2% of all cancers, but approximately 20% of all surgically excised "cold" nodules prove to be cancerous.

The global frequency of palpable and nonpalpable nodules has been evaluated at 4.2% by Wander et al. (1968). The incidence in autopsy series varies from 8% (Schlesinger et al. 1938) to 45.6% (Vidone and Silverberg 1966). The variability of these data makes it almost impossible to determine the true incidence of thyroid cancer. Nevertheless, the high frequency of occult cancers found at autopsy need not obligatorily affect appraisal of the frequency of thyroid malignancies. The apparent rise in the incidence of these cancers may actually be due to the better diagnostic criteria now available for differentiated cancers and the lengthening of the average lifetime which favors an increase in anaplastic cancers. An approximation of 1200 cancers per 1 million population has been proposed (Sancho-Garnier 1977).

The major predisposing factors for thyroid cancers are preexisting thyroid anomalies, age, sex, and a history of prior irradiation (Kendall and Condon 1969; Verby et al. 1969; Williams 1977).

Preexisting thyroid anomalies include goiter, thyroiditis, and hyperthyroidism. Goiter, and especially endemic goiter, was long considered responsible for the increased incidence of thyroid cancer, particularly anaplastic forms, in elderly patients. This classical opinion is today highly debated; it now seems, as suggested by Brown (1981), that the multinodular nature of a goiter considerably reduces, and may even completely annul, the risk of cancer. The frequency of thyroid cancer would thus not exceed 5%, and the risk of malignant change would be practically nil in parenchymatous goiter.

Thyroiditis has also been cited as a predisposing factor. Although associations of cancer and Hashimoto's thyroiditis appear more frequent than would be expected by mere coincidence, not all authors agree as to the existence of a cause-effect relationship. When thyroiditis leads to hypothyroidism, the resulting elevation in TSH may promote carcinogenesis and the development of hormone-dependent follicular or papillary carcinoma.

Hyperthyroidism theoretically prevents the development or progression of thyroid malignancy; those cases reported in the literature are probably the result of mere coincidence or the presence of an occult, sclerosing epithelioma of questionable malignancy (Shapiro et al. 1970).

The patient's age and sex are also important factors affecting the development and prognosis of thyroid cancer (Hirabayashi and Lindsay 1961). Although thyroid malignancies can occur at any age, they are most prevalent in the first two and the last decades, and thyroid cancer is one of the most common malignancies in children and adolescents. Windship and Rosvoll (1961), for example, estimated the risk of cancer at 50% for solitary thyroid nodules in children. Any solitary thyroid nodule in a child or adolescent should thus be considered highly

suspicious for malignancy. By contrast, the majority of anaplastic cancers occur in patients over 60 years of age. The sex distribution usually observed for thyroid pathologies does not apply to thyroid cancers: female predominance is much less marked (sex ratio 2.3), and solitary nodules in young men are thus a cause for suspicion of malignancy.

The third factor warranting consideration is a history of prior irradiation. Several decades ago, cervical radiotherapy was a fairly common procedure for pediatric patients; in the United States of America in particular, it was utilized for a wide variety of conditions ranging from thymic enlargement and cervical adenopathy to neck hemangiomas and even enlarged tonsils and adenoids. Irradiation in adult life involves somewhat different problems; the individuals concerned have either been exposed to radioactive fallout or have received therapeutic radiation for hyperthyroidism. Although it has never been proven conclusively that external beam cervical radiotherapy or administration of radioactive iodine for hyperthyroidism promotes thyroid cancer, it is prudent to reserve radioiodine therapy for patients over 40 years of age.

Familiarity with the etiological characteristics of thyroid cancer better enables the sonographer to provide data which can orient patient management toward surgery or a medical regimen.

2.2.5.2 Thyroid Cancer

Whether occurring alone or concomitantly with a vesicular form, *papillary carcinoma* is the most common malignancy of the thyroid, accounting for 60%–70% of most series. Three-quarters of all patients are females, and it is the most frequent thyroid cancer in young individuals. The prognosis at 10 years is excellent (70%–90% survival). On sonograms, these lesions manifest as generally well-limited, hypoechogenic nodules with multinodular contours (Fig. 2.26). Papillary carcinomas are not compressible when the transducer is pressed down over the corresponding point on the skin, a feature which distinguishes them from adenomas. Intratumoral microcalcifications are visualized as discrete echogenic forms that are too small

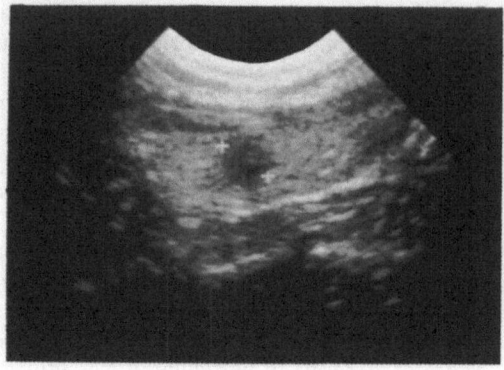

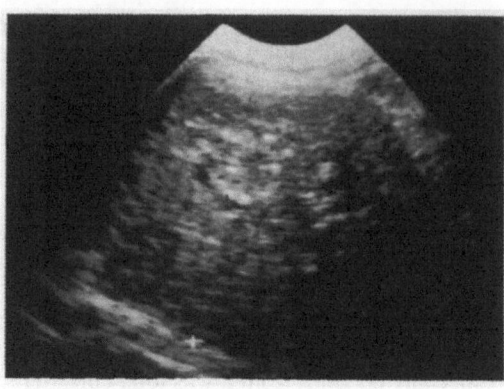

 Fig. 2.26. Small papillary thyroid cancer (7 mm between the two *crosses*)

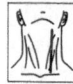 **Fig. 2.27.** Nodule with small, strongly echogenic calcifications without acoustic shadowing (papillary cancer)

to show posterior reinforcement; this can lead to misdiagnosis as a hyperechogenic lesion (Fig. 2.27). Multiple disease foci or micronodules may exist, even at some distance from the main tumor, but they are apt to be small and escape US detection. US can, however, demonstrate the focal nature of lesions, and the absence of perithyroidal involvement. Less often, a papillary tumor manifests sonographically as growths projecting into a cyst from the wall (papillary cystadenocarcinoma). Despite the absence of any ultrasonographic particularities which would allow diagnosis, involvement of the jugulocarotid nodes (Fig. 2.28), and especially subclinical lesions, are frequent with papillary thyroid cancer. The role of the sonographer is to find them, and to suggest the probability of malignancy when a hypoechogenic nodule and adenopathies in the lateral neck are visualized in young patients.

In certain cases, cervical lymphadenopathy predominates both clinically and sonographically. Sonography may fail to detect a small, hypoechogenic thyroid lesion, and the neoplasm will not be diagnosed until the histopathologist has examined the entire homolateral lobectomy specimen.

US is indicated for the follow-up of patients who have undergone total thyroidectomy; local disease recurrence is rare with papillary thyroid cancer, but sonographic exploration can readily demonstrate spread to the jugulocarotid nodes.

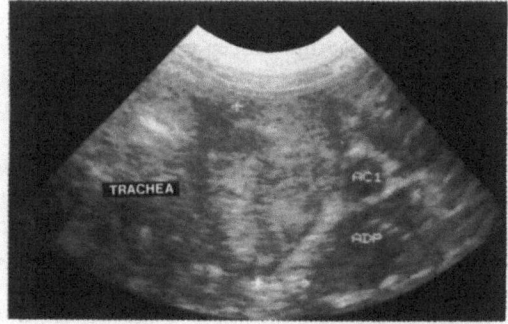

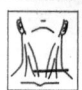 **Fig. 2.28.** Papillary cancer (24 mm between the two *crosses*) with a metastatic retroparotid node *(ADP). AC1,* common carotid artery (transverse scan)

Well-differentiated and moderately differentiated follicular carcinomas account for around 25% of all thyroid cancers (Harness et al. 1984). Well-differentiated follicular cancer is particularly difficult to diagnose, even histologically after fine-needle percutaneous biopsy. The usual diagnosis is adenoma (Figs. 2.29 and 2.30). Even analysis of the surgical specimen may not be conclusive because these solitary, well-encapsulated tumors are composed of more or less dysplastic vesicles resembling normal thyroid tissue or a fetal adenoma. Papillary structure is absent, as are the habitual cytological hallmarks of malignancy. Positive diagnosis is only possible when there are signs of invasion (capsular rupture, vascular involvement).

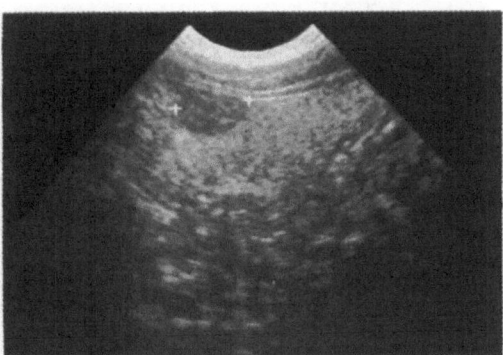

Fig. 2.29. Small, hypoechogenic follicular cancer (12 mm between the two *crosses*)

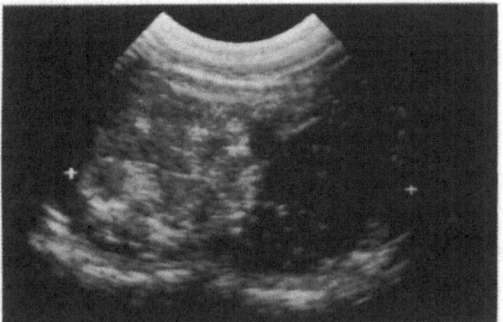

Fig. 2.30. Large thyroid nodule with a complex US pattern (46 mm between the two *crosses*); follicular cancerous tissue is present in the solid component of the nodule

The prognosis for well-differentiated follicular carcinoma is 70% at 10 years. Moderately differentiated follicular carcinoma can also be hard to identify; here again, the only reliable indicators of malignancy are capsular or vascular invasion. The prognosis is slightly less good than for well-differentiated forms (60% at 10 years).

Follicular carcinomas are generally sonographically hypoechogenic and occasionally have a peripheral halo. Hyperechogenic lesions are rare and correspond to well-differentiated forms. Follicular cancer arising in an adenomatous goiter is occasionally diagnosed intra-operatively, but histopathologic examination is generally necessary. US, for example, cannot "pick out" a hypoechogenic lesion in a multi-nodular thyroid with numerous qualitative and quantitative anomalies. Sonographic diagnosis is all the more difficult because follicular cancer characteristically metastasizes via the blood stream, and cervical node involvement is rare.

Undifferentiated (anaplastic) carcinomas represent 15%–20% of all thyroid cancers and can be divided into four histologic forms (giant cell carcinoma, spindle cell carcinoma, small cell carcinoma, mixed or polymorphic carcinoma). Anaplastic carcinomas are highly aggressive, and few patients live longer than 6 months. Clinical diagnosis of these typically large, rapidly growing tumors is fairly easy (cf. Sect. 2.2.1.1). Ultrasonography is useful for confirming the prospective clinical diagnosis because it can distinguish true tumors from enlarged satellite nodes which are frequently mistaken for a tumor on physical examination. Large metastatic nodes often thrombose the internal jugular vein (Figs. 2.31–2.33).

Disease staging is actually best performed with CT, which can also analyze any tracheal or mediastinal involvement. Ultrasound is helpful for determining the best point for percutaneous puncture, a procedure that suffices for diagnosis because of the excellent sensitivity of cytology for this type of cancer. Lesions are often already advanced when diagnosed, and are visualized as more or less diffuse, inhomogeneous images of decreased echogenicity scattered throughout the thyroid gland.

Medullary carcinoma of the thyroid gland arises from the parafollicular C-cells, which secrete thyrocalcitonin and belong to the diffuse endocrine system and APUD (amine precursor uptake and decarboxylation) system. These cells do not concentrate iodine and are not regulated by TSH. The degree of malignancy of medullary thyroid carcinoma is variable; the disease may be hereditary or a component of a multiple endocrine neoplasia (MEN) syndrome. Medullary carcinoma is relatively infrequent, representing only 5% of all thyroid malignancies. As inheritance plays a part in 20%–30% of cases, systematic familial investigations are warranted (Simpson et al. 1982). Medullary tumors vary considerably in size; they are usually solitary except in familial forms and MEN syndromes, which are apt to have multiple disease foci. The presence of amyloid deposits throughout the tumoral stroma

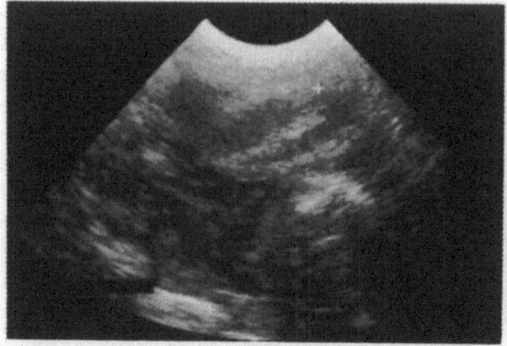

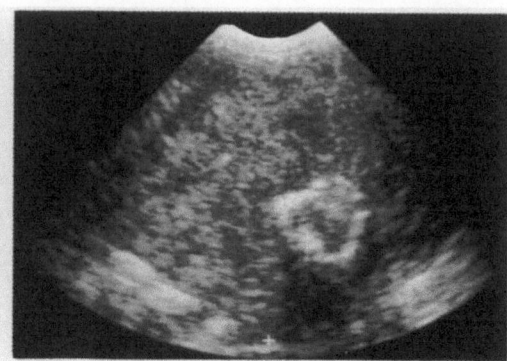

Fig. 2.31. Undifferentiated cancer with a complex US pattern (39 mm between the two *crosses*) (sagittal scan)

Fig. 2.33. Undifferentiated cancer in a goiter: complex US pattern associated with a calcified adenoma (lobe thickness 59 mm)

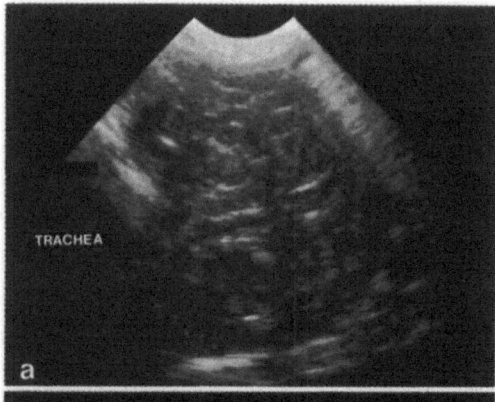

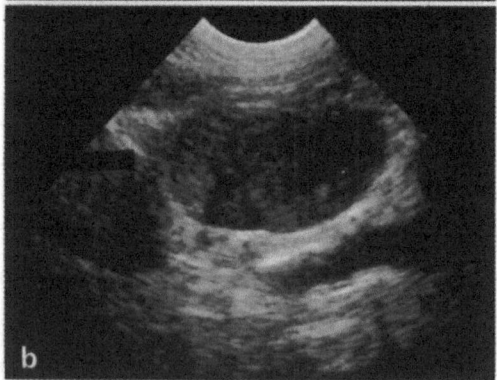

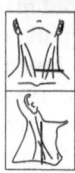
Fig. 2.32 a, b. Undifferentiated thyroid cancer (a) with Metastatic jugular nodes (b)

is characteristic. The three clinical pictures correspond to sporadic forms, familial forms associated with pheochromocytoma, and forms that are part of MEN syndromes. The sporadic form is the most common; it manifests sonographically as an apparently well-limited, hypoechogenic mass, often in the upper third of a thyroid lobe. Compression of the tumor by the transducer may be painful, and the lesion may feel hard. More advanced tumors may invade an entire lobe, which may feel fixed as well as hard (Figs. 2.34 and 2.35). Metastasis to cervical nodes occurs in at least two-thirds of cases.

Careful US evaluation of the liver is also mandatory, because medullary thyroid carcinoma seems to have a predilection for this organ; by contrast, other thyroid tumors rarely metastasize to the liver. Until anatomic proof is obtained, the discovery of hepatic metastases should suggest the possibility of medullary cancer; in most cases there will be advanced lesions. In addition to these clinical and ultrasonographic signs, patients may have watery diarrhea or hot flushes that cease after tumor removal. Diagnosis can be affirmed by assays of the two tumor markers thyrocalcitonin and carcinoembryonic antigen (Calmettes et al. 1979; Tubiana et al. 1968). Discovery of a medullary thyroid cancer should prompt both a familial investigation and a search for pheochromocytoma, which is associated with nearly 10% of medullary thyroid tumors.

Familial medullary thyroid cancer is less frequent than the sporadic form; the tumor is generally diffuse, and involves both thyroid lobes.

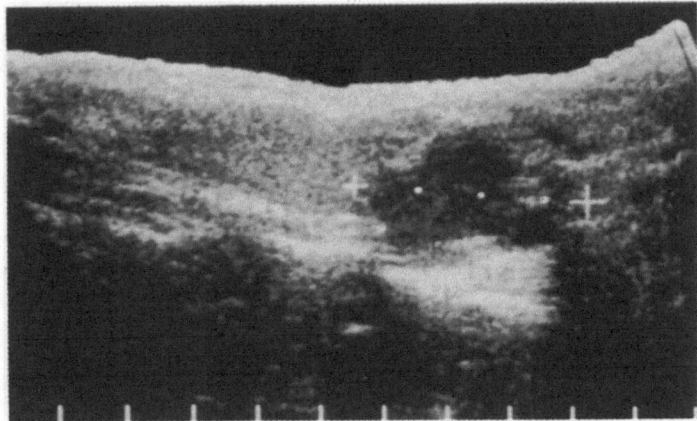

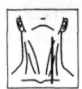
Fig. 2.34. Medullary thyroid cancer (20 mm between the two *crosses*) (sagittal scan)

Association with hyperthyroidism or pheochromocytoma is more common, and thyroid ultrasonography must thus be completed by abdominal US exploration of the adrenal gland region.

Medullary thyroid cancers are occasionally associated with other endocrine disorders or malformations. The most frequent is MEN syndrome type IIa (Sipple's syndrome), an association of characteristically bilateral pheochromocytoma and medullary thyroid carcinoma. Owing to the frequent association of Sipple's syndrome with hyperparathyroidism, ultrasound exploration is more complex: it can demonstrate both thyroid and parathyroid lesions, which may or may not be complicated by jugulocarotid node involvement. The prognosis at 10 years varies from 50%–70%.

Primary and secondary lymphoma of the thyroid are both rare; non-Hodgkin's disease is more common than Hodgkin's disease. Hashimoto's thyroiditis seems to play a predisposing role in the development of thyroid lymphoma. In our experience (Bruneton et al. 1982), thyroid lymphomas can be classed into three sonographic patterns. *Nodules* may at first be mistaken for cystic lesions because of their low echogenicity; the gain setting must be increased to identify their solid nature (Figs. 2.36 and 2.37). Lymphomatous thyroid nodules may be solitary and are often associated with uni- or bilateral lymphomatous nodes of very

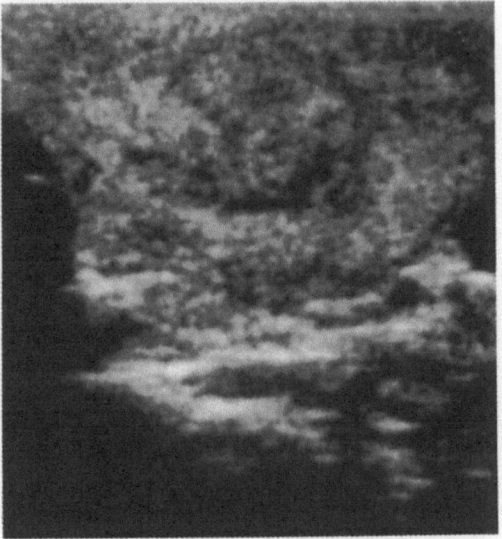

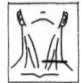
Fig. 2.35. Intraoperative sonogram of a medullary cancer (transverse scan)

decreased echogenicity. Even very large lymphomatous nodes only displace the internal jugular vein, without causing invasion. As emphasized in Chap. 5, such findings are diagnostically important because they suggest lymphoma rather than nodal metastases; once metastases reach a certain size (approximately 5 cm) they thrombose the internal jugular vein,

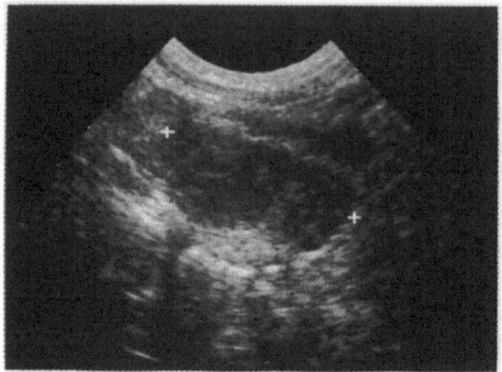

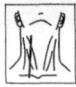
Fig. 2.36. Thyroid lymphoma: gain setting increased so as to fill this very hypoechogenic lesion with echoes (26 mm between the two *crosses*)

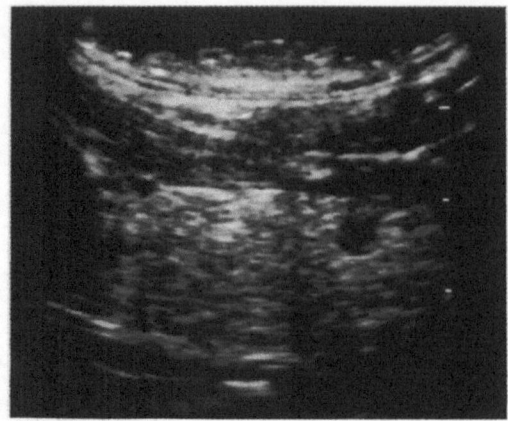

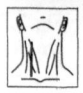
Fig. 2.38. Two thyroid metastases of melanoma (sagittal scan)

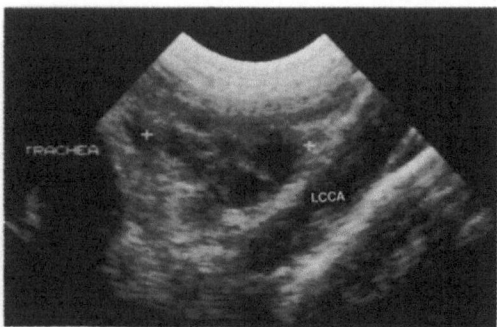

Fig. 2.37. Hypoechogenic pseudoadenomatous nodule in the left thyroid lobe (23 mm between the two *crosses*). The left common carotid artery *(LCCA)* appears horizontal on this transverse scan because this vessel can be very tortuous in elderly patients

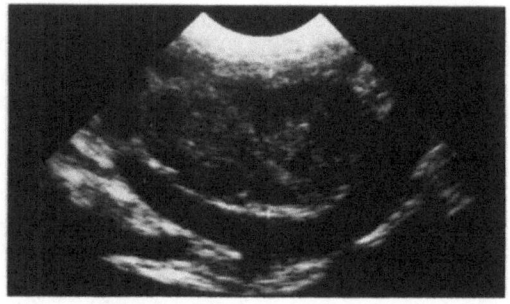

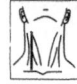
Fig. 2.39. Multiple metastases in the right thyroid lobe of a patient treated for renal cancer (sagittal scan)

whereas lymphomatous nodes of the same dimensions never do.

Diffuse lymphomatous enlargement of the thyroid results in a disorgnaized, complex internal structure similar to that of multinodular goiter. In the absence of any known lymphomatous context, coexistence of cervical lymphadenopathy and a diffusely enlarged thyroid suggests anaplastic carcinoma.

On ultrasound examination, *simple glandular enlargement* due to lymphoma exhibits a normal pattern. Such cases can only be diagnosed retrospectively, when the size of the thyroid decreases along with regression of other lymphomatous lesions in response to chemothera-

py. Accurate measurement of thyroid lobe dimensions is thus mandatory, even if the gland appears normal.

Metastasis to the thyroid is infrequent, occurring late in the course of lung, breast, and kidney cancers, and melanoma (Figs. 2.38 and 2.39), generally as the result of hematogenous spread. Multiple metastatic sites are common. Hypoechogenic nodules of varying size dispersed within healthy thyroid tissue suggest metastasis in a cancer patient with other metastatic sites whose thyroid was normal on a previous sonogram. In practice metastases appear only shortly before death.

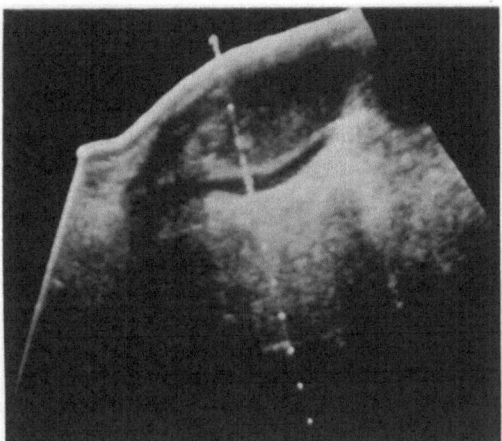

Fig. 2.40. Angiosarcoma of the thyroid

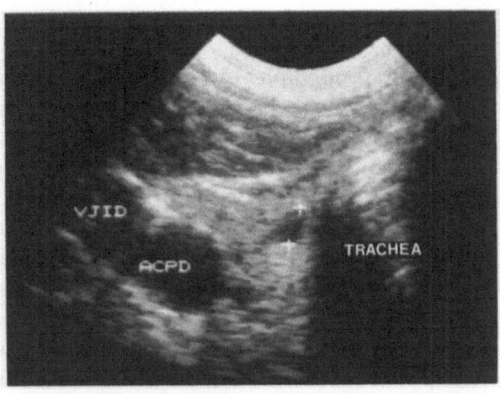

Fig. 2.41. Small solid thyroid lesion followed up by ultrasound during treatment (4 mm between the two *crosses*); return to normal after three months. *VJID*, right internal jugular vein; *ACPD*, right common carotid artery

Thyroid *sarcomas*, including fibrosarcomas, hemangiopericytomas, and angiosarcomas, are also rare. These hypoechogenic lesions characteristically invade an entire thyroid lobe (Fig. 2.40).

2.2.6 Limitations and Potential Improvements of Ultrasonography

2.2.6.1 Thyroid Nodules

Thyroid nodules are rarely the cause of false positive US errors, but care must be taken not to confuse a small adenoma (around 3 mm) with follicular hyperplasia. This anatomic differentiation actually has no practical consequences because these patients are usually left untreated, and at most are followed up by US (Figs. 2.41 and 2.42). False negative errors for the diagnosis of thyroid nodules are also relatively rare; the main cause is a hyper- or hypoechogenic lesion under 5 mm. By contrast, an isoechogenic nodule may not be visualized by US even though it has been palpated clinically. When this occurs, the examination must be repeated with a water bath or Reston interface, and the nodule must be palpated to allow localization. A peripheral halo identifying these lesions is nearly almost always visible.

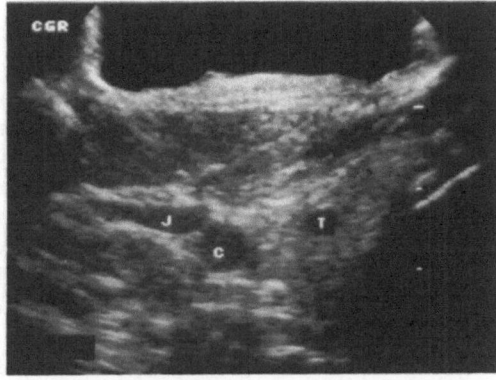

Fig. 2.42. Small, solid thyroid lesion followed up by ultrasonography during treatment. *T*, tumor; *J*, jugular vein; *C*, carotid artery. No modification after 6 months. Examination of the lobectomy specimen disclosed adenoma

Finally, the cystic nature of a lesion containing a thick fluid can prove hard to demonstrate, and the decreased echogenicity may lead to misdiagnosis as a solid lesion.

2.2.6.2 Goiter

While ultrasonography can be used to confirm an already evident clinical diagnosis, its essential role concerns the detection of healthy tissue, in particular at the upper poles of the gland; this point is of major importance for selecting the operative procedure. By contrast, large, often long-standing goiters have a complex US structure, in which solid zones coexist with fluid-filled areas secondary to hemorrhagic necrosis or cystic degeneration. US is incapable of demonstrating focal malignant changes within such goiters. Furthermore, aside from clinical signs of progressive disease or the presence of cervical lymphadenopathy, the US appearance of adenomatous goiter is nearly the same as that of an undifferentiated carcinoma.

2.2.6.3 Potential Improvements in Thyroid Sonography

Future improvements in the utility of US for thyroid studies will rely on two different techniques. The first, fine-needle aspiration biopsy, is already employed in numerous countries and has proven truly effective. Although an asymptomatic thyroid nodule may be left untreated and merely kept under surveillance, the high sensitivity of fine-needle aspiration biopsy and its low degree of invasiveness warrant use on a wider scale, even though only a positive result is valid for a diagnosis of malignancy. Chapter 1 mentioned recent reports on ultrasound-directed punctures using certain transducers and special needles. This simple technique currently appears feasible for thyroid nodules of 5-10 mm, meaning that many patients can rapidly be reassured as to their condition. The second potential improvement concerns tissue characterization by sonographic procedures, most likely in conjunction with radiofrequency waveform analysis (Benson et al. 1983). This technique is noninvasive but necessitates larger, more complex apparatus than US equipment. Results obtained to date are promising, but are still no better than percutaneous fine-needle puncture biopsy.

2.2.7 Protocol for the Exploration of Thyroid Nodules

For tumoral pathologies, ultrasound is currently indicated for determination of the number of nodules in a thyroid (so that the best therapeutic solution can be adopted), search for a primary tumor, and, if there is a history of previous cervical irradiation, possibly tumor diagnosis (Simeone et al. 1982).

Owing to its high anatomic sensitivity for nodule detection, ultrasonography is unquestionably the first examination warranted after physical examination. In our experience, the sensitivities of intraoperative US and intraoperative palpation are comparable; the operative procedure can therefore reliably be based on ultrasound data (Bruneton et al. 1985). As an illustration, a negative sonogram for the lobe contralateral to a thyroid lesion obviates the need for systematic surgical exploration of this lobe. By contrast, if surgery has been decided upon, the surgeon should remove a nodule contralateral to one or more thyroid lesions in a thyroid lobe. Nodules smaller than 7 mm in the midportion of a lobe may not be palpable. Intraoperative ultrasonography is particularly helpful for the surgeon in these cases because lesion localization allows enucleation. Again, US detection of neoplastic foci is impossible in cases of adenomatous thyroid enlargement; diagnosis is possible only by histological examination of the thyroidectomy specimen. For Brown (1981), however, solitary

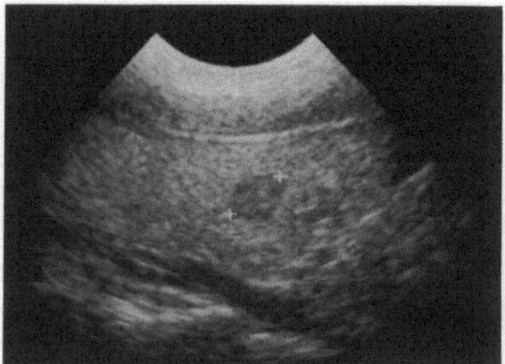

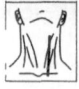 **Fig. 2.43.** Small hypoechogenic thyroid nodule corresponding to a papillary cancer (8 mm between the two *crosses*)

nodules have more chance of being malignant (10%–20% of cases) than multinodular lesions (1%–6%).

Although US cannot differentiate carcinoma from adenoma any more than other imaging methods (Kendall and Condon 1969), hyperechogenic and extremely necrotic nodules as well as multiple lesions tend to suggest a benign process. By contrast, solitary nodules, dominant metastatic disease, a history of prior cervical irradiation, and concomitant cervical node involvement are all factors justifying immediate surgery, regardless of lesion size on sonograms (Fig. 2.43).

For patients followed up during treatment, ultrasound is a valuable means of monitoring response, as reflected by modifications in the size or sonographic appearance of lesions.

2.3 Thyroiditis

Roughly speaking, thyroiditis can be divided into several different categories:

- acute and subacute: acute bacterial thyroiditis, pseudotuberculous thyroiditis, de Quervain's giant cell thyroiditis
- chronic lymphocytic thyroiditis without associated autoimmune disease: tuberculous or syphilitic thyroiditis, Riedel's nonspecific thyroiditis, nonspecific giant cell thyroiditis, nonspecific thyroiditis in conjunction with a nodular goiter
- chronic lymphocytic thyroiditis with signs of autoimmune disease: diffuse form in a hypertrophic gland or Hashimoto's thyroiditis, diffuse form in an atrophic gland during myxedema, diffuse or focal form in a normal gland during asymptomatic thyroiditis, focal form in a nodular goiter or thyroid cancer, focal or diffuse form in a toxic goiter

The actual implications of thyroiditis vary with the form. For certain etiologies, such as cancer, coexisting thyroiditis is merely of physiopathological interest. Acute bacterial thyroiditis is rarely encountered today and can generally be linked to local thyroid infection secondary to septicemia. The poorly delimited, hypoechogenic zone first visualized by US will be found on further examination to actually correspond to a central anechogenic area with possibly

thick walls. Patterns of this sort can resemble a necrotic adenoma, but lesions are apt to enlarge rapidly if there is a febrile context, and passage of the transducer over the neck is painful. In actuality, the diagnosis is made clinically, and US is merely a confirmatory procedure.

Sonographic exploration is essentially limited to the workup of four major forms: de Quervain's thyroiditis, Hashimoto's thyroiditis, Riedel's thyroiditis, and strumitis or thyroiditis affecting a preexisting goiter.

2.3.1 De Quervain's Subacute Thyroiditis

This pathology is often characterized by a generalized, acute phase of thyroid inflammation

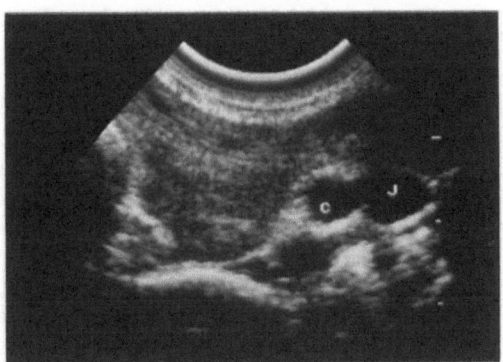

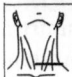
Fig. 2.44. Inhomogeneous decreased echogenicity of the thyroid gland in subacute thyroiditis. *C*, primary carotid artery; *J*, internal jugular vein (transverse scan)

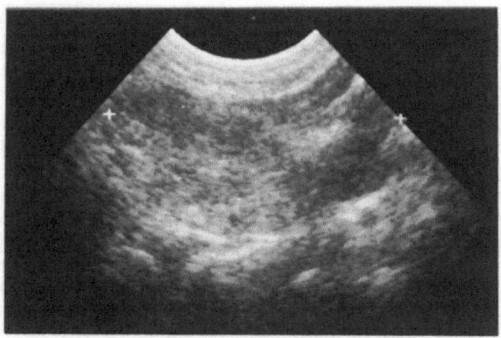

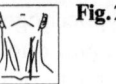
Fig. 2.45. Subacute thyroiditis (sagittal scan)

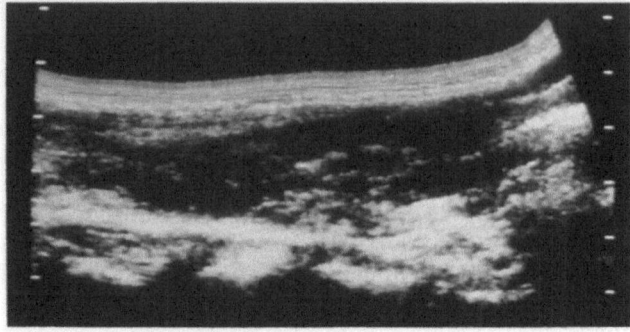

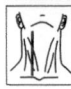 **Fig. 2.46.** Hashimoto's thyroiditis (sagittal scan)

together with asthenia, fever, and muscular pain, often shortly after an upper respiratory tract infection or at the same time as a viral disease. The thyroid feels firm, with a bosselated surface and a nodular consistency; the covering skin feels warm; satellite node involvement is possible (Greene 1971). The sedimentation rate is typically high. The isotope uptake pattern on thyroid scintiscans may be patchy or negligible. Transition between these often focal hypoechogenic lesions and normal tissue is progressive (Blum et al. 1977; Espinasse 1983; Poncin and Hassan, 1983). Lesions tend to be bilateral rather than unilateral, and US data plus clinical signs allow diagnosis (Figs. 2.44 and 2.45).

The disease responds favorably to administration of corticosteroids or common anti-inflammatory drugs, and the US images return to normal. Nodular transformation of focal disease is a rare possibility, however, and a repeat sonogram should be obtained after the acute inflammatory crisis has subsided.

2.3.2 Hashimoto's Thyroiditis

Hashimoto's thyroiditis usually presents in women between the third and sixth decades. The thyroid is usually moderately enlarged, causing vague neck pain, and the patient is euthyroid. The thyroid gland is firm, with a bosselated surface. Ultrasonography confirms enlargement of the gland; thyroid hypoechogenicity is an almost constant feature, and once it occurs seems durable. The echogenicity of the gland may be as low as that of the adjacent muscles, and in particular the sternocleidomastoid muscle. Aside from Hashimoto's thyroiditis, the only affection in which this same pattern is seen is Graves' disease, but this last pathology occurs in an entirely different context (Fig. 2.46). Hashimoto's thyroiditis can therefore be diagnosed before the constantly high antimicrosomial and antithyroglobulin antibody titers associated with this pathology are found (Bastanie and Roitt 1972). Thyroid scintiscans may or may not be uniform. On US examination, the cold zones seen on scintiscans are visualized as nodules of increased echogenicity relative to the globally hypoechogenic gland.

The frequency of cold nodules varies from 10%–50% (Espinasse 1983; Simeone et al. 1982). The goiter responds favorably to treatment and regresses in size; the disease runs a chronic course, however, and its US pattern changes little with time. Although the fact has no sonographic implications, Hashimoto's thyroiditis tends to be latent rather than clinically overt. According to Gordin et al. (1979) 2%–5% of all euthyroid individuals are positive for antithyroid antibodies and have elevated TSH levels.

2.3.3 Riedel's Thyroiditis
(Invasive Fibrous Thyroiditis)

Riedel's struma, as it is also called, is an exceedingly rare condition characterized by a stony-hard gland and extension into surround-

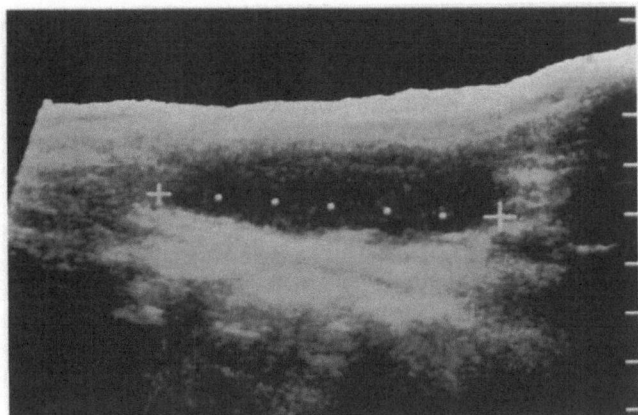

Fig. 2.47. Riedel's thyroiditis (sagittal scan)

ing structures that can cause often severe compression (Woolner et al. 1957). Whether focal or scattered throughout the thyroid, the hypoechogenic tumoral masses visualized by US resist compression by the transducer (Fig. 2.47).

The preoperative diagnosis is thus usually cancer; surgical exploration is required to identify it correctly. There is no medical treatment, and surgery is the only useful therapy. Postoperative disease recurrence is rare. Certain studies have emphasized the association between this rare type of thyroiditis and retroperitoneal fibrosis.

2.3.4 Strumitis on Goiter

This condition is also quite rare, and the development of hypoechogenic zones within a multinodular goiter may suggest malignant transformation to an anaplastic cancer, especially if the inflammatory syndrome is not very severe. Both clinical and US findings point towards malignancy, and the true diagnosis requires surgery.

2.4 Thyroid Dysfunction

2.4.1 Hyperthyroidism

Hyperthyroidism has various origins, including Graves' disease (the most frequent cause), adenoma, and multinodular toxic goiter. Other possible etiologies (thyrotoxic thyroiditis, exogenous hyperthyroidism due to ectopic secretion of thyroid hormones, or excessive TSH secretion) are much rarer and are not described further.

2.4.1.1 Graves' Disease

The autoimmune etiology of Graves' disease has been demonstrated by the presence of classical autoantibodies (such as automicrosomial antibodies) during the course of the disease; the most specific antibodies are the circulating TSH receptor antibodies and long-acting thyroid stimulator (Knox et al. 1976; Labhart 1974). Other antibodies have also been evidenced (TSI, TDI, TGI); these immunoglobulins, directed against TSH receptors, reproduce the different effects of TSH. Graves' disease appears to result from disruption of the balance of the immune system, leading to the production of thyroid-stimulating immunoglobulins causing thyrotoxicosis, goiter, and ophthalmopathy. The best example of the factor causing this imbalance is stress in individuals

with an inherited predisposition (Volpe 1978).
The clinical picture of Graves' disease is variable, but it classically associates goiter, ocular
manifestations, and pretibial myxedema.

The goiter is habitually diffuse, rubbery, homogeneous, symmetrical, and nontender; the cervical lymph nodes are usually not involved. A
thrill and a murmur may be heard at auscultation, particularly over the upper pole of the thyroid lobes. The thyroid gland generally appears
enlarged on sonograms, even though Poncin-
Viateau and Hassan (1985) reported a normal
thyroid volume in 20% of patients. The echogenicity of the gland is not as low as in Hashimoto's thyroiditis and is occasionally hard to
detect. The degree of hypoechogenicity is not
related to the clinical or biological stage of the
disease. In addition to moderately hypoechogenic forms, the thyroid may also appear inhomogeneous and present lobulations smaller
than 1 cm in greatest dimension; the resultant
pseudonodular appearance should not be confused with adenomatous goiter. The thyroid
gland of patients with Grave's disease is rarely
sonographically normal (Figs. 2.48 and 2.49).
Along with analysis of the goiter, US is indicated for monitoring the extent and evolution of
the concomitant ophthalmopathy. The diagnosis is made clinically and affirmed by the elevated levels of T_3 and T_4; the TSH is normal or
decreased.

When radioiodine treatment is envisaged, sonographic evaluation of gland volume is a useful
means of selecting the appropriate dose (cf.
Chap. 1). After radioiodine treatment the thyroid regresses in size and atrophies, becoming
inhomogeneously hyperechogenic (Poncin-
Viateau and Hassan 1985).

2.4.1.2 Toxic Adenoma

The estimated incidence of toxic adenoma
varies from 17%–70%. These always solitary lesions typically arise in the otherwise normal
thyroid of a woman, and should be considered
benign tumors. Cardiac symptoms (auricular
fibrillation, tachycardia with or without cardiac
insufficiency) often predominate (Hamburger
1975).

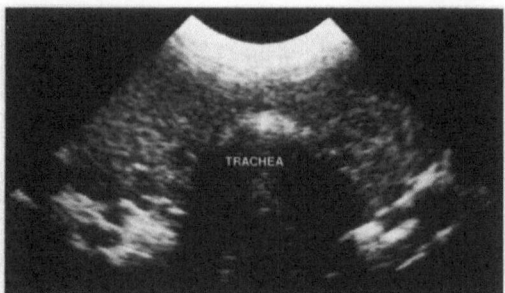

Fig. 2.48. Moderate thyroid enlargement in
a patient with Graves' disease (transverse
scan)

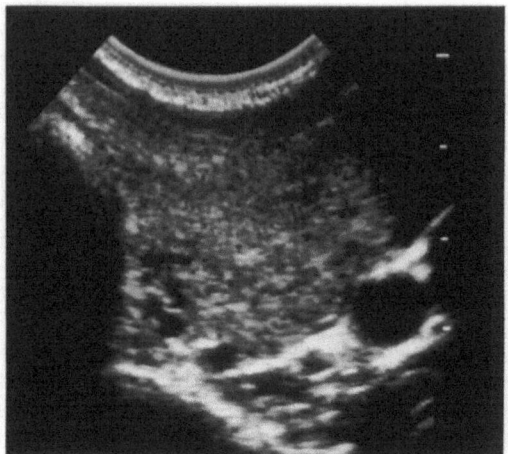
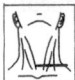

Fig. 2.49. Transverse scan of the left thyroid
lobe in a patient with Graves' disease; the
rounded and linear images are dilated intrathyroid veins

The sonographic patterns of toxic adenomas
are quite variable (hypoechogenic, cystic, or
even hyperechogenic). Above all, US can demonstrate whether or not the contralateral lobe is
normal; radionuclide scanning cannot provide
this information because elective radioactive
tracer uptake by the nodule prevents visualization of the adjacent and contralateral thyroid
parenchyma.

Toxic adenoma is similar to toxic multinodular
goiter, a frequent cause of hyperthyroidism of
late onset in patients with multinodular goiter.
Toxic multinodular goiter is thus essentially a
geriatric pathology. Cardiovascular distur-
bances are usually severe. US will visualize a

multinodular gland, but cannot identify the toxic nodule; this information is provided by scintigraphy.

2.4.2 Hypothyroidism

2.4.2.1 Primary Hypothyroidism

Primary hypothyroidism, the most frequent form, is generally secondary to an anatomic lesion, associated (or not) with gland dysfunction. It essentially affects elderly women. Thyroid dysgenesis, including thyroid ectopia (Neimann et al. 1968), athyreosis, and congenital dyshormonogenesis, is rare in children. Acquired hormonopoietic disorders are usually caused by abusive use of synthetic antithyroid drugs. Iatrogenic destruction of the thyroid can also lead to acquired primary hypothyroidism. Thyroid surgery is the major cause, and both total thyroidectomy (after which hypothyroidism can be prevented by systemic administration of hormones) and subtotal thyroidectomy (in which a functioning piece of thyroid is left in place to ensure euthyroidism) have been implicated (MacNeil and Thomson 1968). Hypothyroidism, though often moderate, has been estimated to occur in nearly 10% of patients after thyroidectomy.

Another cause of hypothyroidism is treatment with certain radioisotopes (particularly iodine-131), which accounts for over 25% of cases. Thyroiditis, and especially Hashimoto's thyroiditis, may be associated with or lead to hypothyroidism.

Primary hypothyroidism is the most important cause of spontaneous myxedema in adults. The diffuse, bilateral atrophy of the gland demonstrated sonographically is associated with a massive elevation in circulating antithyroid antibody concentrations.

2.4.2.2 Secondary Hypothyroidism

Secondary hypothyroidism is due to insufficient thyrotropin secretion. Diagnosis is based on an adequate thyroid response to exogenous TSH and a decreased plasma TSH level. There is usually a more or less complete context of hypopituitarism; the main etiology is pituitary

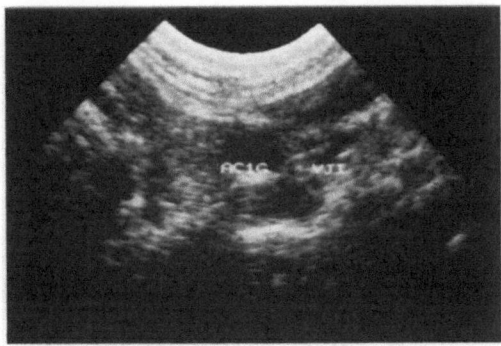

Fig. 2.50. Small thyroid lobe in a hypothyroid patient. *ACIG,* left common carotid artery; *VJI,* internal jugular vein (transverse scan)

adenoma. Here again, the thyroid appears atrophic on sonograms (Fig. 2.50).

2.5 The Postsurgery Thyroid

Thyroid surgery makes use of a variety of operative procedures: simple enucleation, loboisthmectomy, and subtotal or total thyroidectomy, completed (or not) by node dissection (Fig. 2.51). Enucleation scars are not visible sonographically.

After uni- or bilateral loboisthmectomy, the laterotracheal region is only weakly echogenic; above all, the common carotid artery and the internal jugular vein occupy very medial locations, almost applied against the larynx and trachea (Figs. 2.52 and 2.53). After loboisthmectomy or lobectomy for adenoma (Fig. 2.54), the condition of the remaining thyroid tissue can be evaluated by US. Along with providing volumetric data, sonography will reveal any new adenomatous lesions.

Cervical ultrasonography is particularly important for the follow-up of patients who have undergone surgery for thyroid cancer. After subtotal thyroidectomy, US can evaluate the remaining thyroid tissue (Christensen et al. 1983). After total thyroidectomy, it can explore the laterotracheal regions for possible disease recurrence (Jacobs et al. 1983). Thyroid sonography must be completed by exploration of the jugulocarotid lymph node chains to detect any late sites of metastasis.

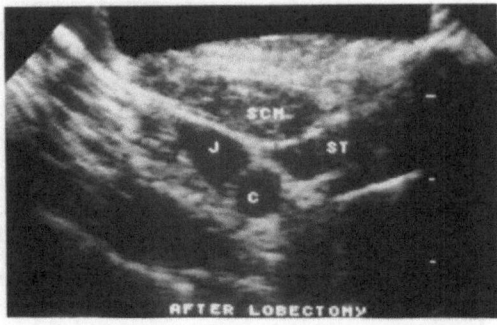

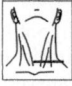 **Fig. 2.51.** Cervical hematoma after lobecto-my (43 mm between the two *crosses*). *AC1G*, left common carotid artery; *VJIG*, left internal jugular vein (transverse scan)

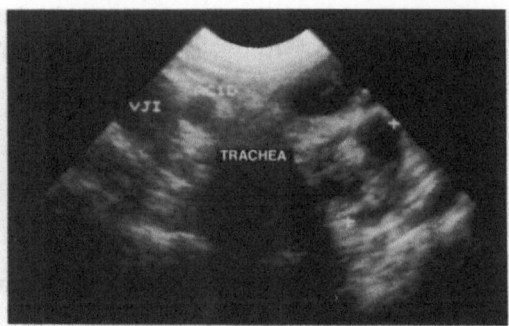

 Fig. 2.53. Normal transverse scan after total thyroidectomy. *C*, common carotid artery; *J*, internal jugular vein; *T*, trachea

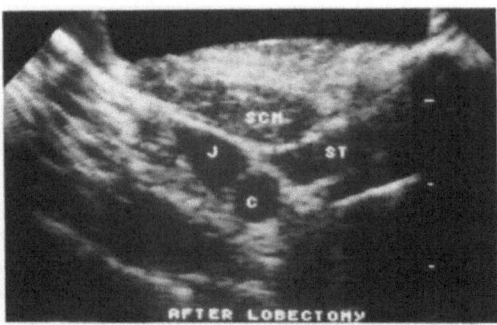

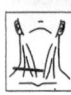 **Fig. 2.52.** Normal transverse scan after lo-bectomy. *J*, internal jugular vein; *C*, common carotid artery; *SCM*, sternocleidomas-toid muscle; *ST*, sternothyroid muscle

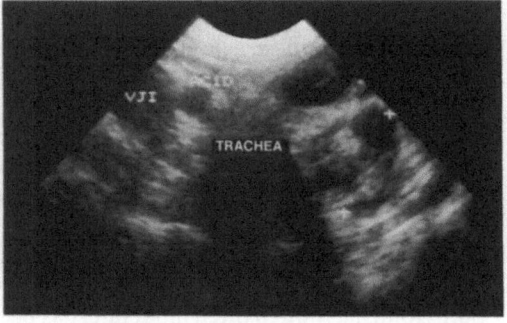

 Fig. 2.54. Adenoma in the remaining lobe after right lobectomy (21 mm between the two *crosses*); the right common carotid artery *(AC1D)* and the internal jugular vein *(VJI)* can be seen medially (transverse scan)

2.6 References

Allen FH, Krook PM, De Groot WPH (1979) Ultrasound demonstration of a thyroid carcinoma within a benign cyst. AJR 132: 136–137

Bastanie PA, Roitt IM (1972) Thyroiditis and thyroid function. Pergamon, Oxford

Beckers C (1979) Thyroid nodules. Clin Endocrinol Metab 8: 181–192

Benson DM, Rifkin MD, Rose JL, Goldberg BB (1983) Characterization of benign and malignant tissues of the thyroid gland. An ultrasonic approach using RF waveform analysis and pattern recognition. Invest Radiol 18: 459–462

Block MA, Dailey GE, Robb JA (1983) Thyroid nodules indeterminate by needle biopsy. Am J Surg 146: 72–76

Blum M, Passalaqua AM, Sackler JP, Pudlowski M (1977) Thyroid echography of subacute thyroiditis. Radiology 125: 795–798

Brown CL (1981) Pathology of the cold nodule. Clin Endocrinol Metab 10: 235–245

Bruneton JN, Caramella E (1984) Tumeurs de la thyroïde. In: Bruneton JN, Matter D, Benozio M, Senecail B (eds) Echographie en pathologie tumorale de l'adulte. Masson, Paris, pp 1–6

Bruneton JN, Caramella E, Boublil JL, Roux P, Abbes M, Demard F (1982) Echographic aspects of thyroid and parotid localizations in non-Hodgkin's lymphomas. Rofo 136: 530–533

Bruneton JN, Caramella E, Fenart D, Ettore F, Manzino JJ, Demard F, Vallicioni J (1985) Echographie ultrasonore en temps réel de haute définition des tumeurs du corps thyroïde. A propos de 379 cas opérés. J Radiol 66: 59–63

Calmettes C, Mouktar MS, Milhaud G (1979) Calcitonine et antigène carcino-embryonnaire: marqueurs tumoraux au cours du cancer médullaire de la thyroïde. Nouv Presse Med 8: 3947–3950

Carroll BA (1982) Asymptomatic thyroid nodules: incidental sonographic detection. AJR 133: 499–501

Christensen SB, Ljungberg O, Tibblin S (1983) Surgical treatment of thyroid carcinoma in a defined population: 1960 to 1977. Evaluation of the results after a conservative surgical approach. Am J Surg 146: 349–354

Cole-Beuglet C, Goldberg BB (1983) New high-resolution ultrasound evaluation of diseases of the thyroid gland. A review article. JAMA 249: 2941–2944

Espinasse P (1983) L'échographie thyroïdienne dans les thyroïdites lymphocytaires chroniques autoimmunes. J Radiol 64: 537–544

Gerard-Marchand R (1977) The classification of thyroid cancers according to the TNM system. Ann Radiol 20: 700–702

Glazer GM, Axel L, Moss AA (1982) CT diagnosis of mediastinal thyroid. AJR 138: 495–498

Gordin A, Maatela J, Miettinen A, Helenius T, Lamberg BA (1979) Serum thyrotrophin and circulating thyroglobulin and thyroid microsomial antibodies in a population. Acta Endocrinol (Copenh) 90: 33–42

Greene JN (1971) Subacute thyroiditis. Am J Med 51: 97–108

Greening WP, Sarker SK, Osborne MP (1980) Hemiagenesis of the thyroid gland. Br J Surg 67: 446–448

Hamburger JI (1975) Solitary autonomously functioning thyroid lesions. Diagnosis, clinical features, and pathogenetic considerations. Am J Med 58: 740–748

Harness JK, Thompson NW, McLeod MK, Eckhauser FE, Lloyd RV (1984) Follicular carcinoma of the thyroid gland: trends and treatment. Surgery 96: 972–980

Heim M, Chrestian M, Henry JF, Van Lidt H, Vidal D, Simonin R (1984) Nodules thyroïdiens. Valeur diagnostique de la cytoponction à l'aiguille fine. Cent cinquante-neuf malades opérés. Presse Med 13: 1369–1372

Hirabayashi RN, Lindsay S (1961) Carcinoma of the thyroid. A statistical study of 390 patients. J Clin Endocrinol 21: 1596–1610

Jacobs JK, Aland JW Jr, Ballinger JF (1983) Total thyroidectomy. A review of 213 patients. Ann Surg 197: 542–548

Jennings AS, Atkinson BF (1983) Thyroid needle aspiration: collecting and handling the specimen. New Engl J Med 308: 1602–1603

Katz JF, Kane RA, Reyes J, Clarke MP, Hill TC (1984) Thyroid nodules: sonographic-pathologic correlation. Radiology 151: 741–745

Kendall LW, Condon RE (1969) Prediction of malignancy in solitary thyroid nodules. Lancet 1: 1071–1073

Knox AJ, Von Westarp C, Row VV, Volpe R (1976) Thyroid antigen stimulates lymphocytes from patients with Graves' disease to produce thyroid-stimulating immunoglobulins (TSI). J Clin Endocrinol Metab 43: 330–337

Labhart A (1974) Clinical endocrinology. Springer, Berlin Heidelberg New York

Leopold GR (1980) Ultrasonography of superficially located structures. Radiol Clin North Am 18: 161–173

Lo Gerfo P, Colacchio T, Caushaj F, Weber C, Feind C (1982) Comparison of fine-needle and coarse-needle biopsies in evaluating thyroid nodules. Surgery 92: 835–838

MacNeil AD, Thomson JA (1968) Long term follow up of surgically treated thyrotoxic patients. Br Med J 3: 643–646

Mazzaferri EL (1981) Solitary thyroid nodule: selective approach to management. Postgrad Med 70: 107–109

Miller JM, Hamburger JI, Kini SR (1981) The needle biopsy diagnosis of papillary thyroid carcinoma. Cancer 48: 989–993

Moreau JF, Carlier-Conrads L (eds) (1984) Imagerie diagnostique des glandes thyroïde et parathyroïdes. Vigot, Paris

Neimann N, Pierson M, Martin J, Sapelier J (1968) L'ectopie de la thyroïde, cause principale de l'hypothyroïdie infantile. Presse Med 76: 659–663

Pacini F, Pinchera A, Giani C, Grasso L, Doveri F, Bascheri L (1980) Serum thyroglobulin in thyroid carcinoma and other thyroid disorders. J Endocrinol Invest 3: 238–292

Poncin J, Hassan M (1983) Echographie des thyroïdites non suppurées. J Radiol 64: 713–720

Poncin-Viateau J, Hassan M (1985) Echographie thyroïdienne. Vigot, Paris, pp 87–103

Prinz RA, O'Morchoe PJ, Barbato AL, Braithwaite SS, Brooks MH, Emanuele MA, Lawrence AM, Paloyan E (1983) Fine needle aspiration biopsy of thyroid nodules. Ann Surg 198: 70–73

Radecki PD, Arger PH, Avenson RL, Jennings AS, Coleman BG, Mintz MC, Kressel HY (1984) Thyroid imaging: comparison of high-resolution real time ultrasound and computed tomography. Radiology 153: 145–147

Sancho-Garnier H (1977) Epidemiology of thyroid cancer. Ann Radiol 20: 715–721

Scheible W, Leopold GR, Woo VL, Gosink BB (1979) High-resolution real-time ultrasonography of thyroid nodules. Radiology 133: 413–417

Schlesinger MJ, Gargill SL, Saxe IH (1938) Studies in nodular goiter: incidence of thyroid nodules in routine necropsies in a nongoitrous region. JAMA 110: 1638–1641

Schlumberger M, Fragu P, Parmentier C, Tubiana M (1981) Thyroglobulin assay in the follow-up of patients with differentiated thyroid carcinomas: comparison of its value in patients with or without normal residual tissue. Acta Endocrinol (Copenh) 98: 215–221

Shapiro SJ, Friedmann NB, Perzik SL, Catz B (1970) Incidence of thyroid carcinoma in Graves' disease. Cancer 26: 1261-1270

Silverman PM, Newman GE, Korobkin M, Workman JB, Moore AV, Coleman RE (1984) Computed tomography in the evaluation of thyroid disease. AJR 141: 897-902

Simeone JF, Daniels GH, Mueller PR, Maloof F, Van Sonnenberg E, Hall DA, O'Connell RS, Ferucci JT Jr, Wittenberg J (1982) High-resolution real-time sonography of the thyroid. Radiology 145: 431-435

Simpson WJ, Palmer JA, Rosen IB, Mustard RA (1982) Management of medullary carcinoma of the thyroid. Am J Surg 144: 420-422

Solbiati L, Volterrani L, Rizzatto G, Bazzocchi M, Busilacchi P, Candiani F, Ferrari F, Giuseppetti G, Maresca G, Mirk P, Rubaltelli L, Zappasodi F (1985) The thyroid gland with low uptake lesions: evaluation by ultrasound. Radiology 155: 187-191

Stark DD, Clark OH, Gooding GA, Moss AA (1983) High-resolution ultrasonography and computed tomography of thyroid lesions in patients with hyperparathyroidism. Surgery 94: 863-868

Tubiana M, Milhaud G, Lacour J (1968) Medullary carcinoma and thyrocalcitonin. Br Med J 4: 87-89

Verby JE, Woolner LB, Nobrega T, Kurland LT, McConahey WM (1968) Thyroid cancer in Olmsted County (1935-1965). J Nat Cancer Inst 43: 813-820

Vidone RA, Silverberg SG (1966) Carcinoma of the thyroid in surgical and postmortem material. Ann Surg 164: 291-299

Volpe R (1978) The pathogenesis of Graves' disease: an overview. J Clin Endocrinol Metab 7: 3-29

Wander JB, Gaston EA, Dawber TR (1968) The significance of non-toxic nodules. Ann Intern Med 69: 537-540

Williams ED (1977) The epidemiology of thyroid cancer. Ann Radiol 20: 722-724

Windship T, Rosvoll RV (1961) Childhood thyroid cancer. Am J Surg 102: 747-752

Woolner LB, McConahey WM, Beahrs OH (1957) Invasive fibrous thyroiditis (Riedel's struma). J Clin Endocrinol Metab 17: 201-220

3 Parathyroid Glands

J.-F. MOREAU

The principal indication for ultrasonography of the parathyroid glands is exploration of tumoral lesions secondary to hyperparathyroidism. Hypoparathyroidism, which can result in tetany, cannot be evaluated by imaging techniques and particularly not by ultrasonography (US), and there are no inflammatory or infectious pathologies. Hyperparathyroidism detected by an elevated serum parathyroid level is generally managed by surgery, except when contraindicated by the patient's age or general condition. Both primary and secondary hyperparathyroidism involve well-known surgical difficulties, and while an experienced parathyroid surgeon may feel confident enough to proceed without having recourse to imaging techniques, the value of the preoperative information they provide is increasingly apparent. This is particularly true for US, even though sonographic data alone are insufficient for diagnostic purposes.

3.1 General Features of Hyperparathyroidism

The parathyroid glands play an essential role in maintaining a constant calcium ion concentration. The conjoined actions of parathyroid hormone (PTH), secreted by the parathyroid glands, on bone, the kidneys, and the gastrointestinal tract are responsible for elevating the calcium level. In bone PTH stimulates the activity of the preexisting osteoclasts, activates periosteocytic osteolysis, and rapidly inhibits the metabolic activity of the osteoclasts. In the kidney PTH promotes urinary excretion of phosphate and bicarbonate, and enhances renal tubular reabsorption of calcium. In the intestine PTH accelerates gastrointestinal absorption of calcium in synergy with vitamin D. Three forms of hyperparathyroidism have been defined: primary, secondary, and tertiary.

3.1.1 Primary Hyperparathyroidism

Primary hyperparathyroidism is caused by excess PTH secretion by an adenoma, hyperplasia, or carcinoma of a parathyroid gland or glands. Contrary to a formerly held opinion, it is a fairly common disorder whose incidence has increased over the past 10 years, although this is probably due to routine screening for hypercalcemia rather than to a true increase in the frequency of the disease. For Boonstra and Jackson (1965) routine biochemical screening detected hypercalcemia in the absence of clinical symptoms in 1 case per 1000 population, and about 80% of cases were related to hyperparathyroidism. There is a marked female predominance (sex ratio 2:1), and although it can occur at any age, most patients are over 40 years of age.

3.1.1.1 Clinical Presentation

The wide range of reliable biochemical tests, the ease with which serum PTH can be measured, and the unquestionable benefits provided by imaging techniques, in particular US, all explain why primary hyperparathyroidism is increasingly associated with only vague clinical symptoms. Today, hyperparathyroidism is considered a possibility not only for patients with urinary tract or bone manifestations, but also for those with otherwise unexplained asthenia, weight loss, or gastrointestinal symptoms (abdominal pain, nausea, constipation). The classical clinical picture of hyperparathyroidism involves a combination of bone, renal, gastrointestinal, cardiovascular, and psychoneurologic manifestations. It is often incomplete at diagnosis, with only one or several of the clinical features cited hereafter present.

Bone lesions can include osteitis fibrosa cystica accompanied by bone pain, bone swelling, and/or spontaneous fracture. Both extensive skeletal demineralization and focal resorption can be demonstrated radiologically. The sclerotic changes of osteosclerosis almost always observed in secondary hyperparathyroidism are less frequent in primary hyperparathyroidism. Urolithiasis represents the major renal manifestation and occurs in 50%–80% of patients with hyperparathyroidism. Inversely, according to Black and Haff (1970), hyperparathyroidism is associated with only about 5% of all cases of lithiasis; the incidence rises to 12%–15% for patients with recurrent lithiasis. Nephrocalcinosis and chronic renal insufficiency are infrequent. Gastrointestinal manifestations are dominated by functional signs: abdominal pain, nausea, vomiting, anorexia, constipation. Peptic ulcers tend to be duodenal rather than gastric and occur in 10%–20% of cases. Pancreatitis is uncommon. Cardiovascular manifestations are secondary to arterial hypertension, which may be due to renal disease or merely the result of hypercalcemia. Psychoneurologic manifestations can include a combination of asthenia, muscular weakness, hypotonia, and chronic or acute mental disorders.

3.1.1.2 Diagnosis

As determined by biochemical tests, hypercalcemia usually ranges from 110–130 mg/liter; there may be associated hypophosphatemia, hypercalciuria, and/or hyperphosphaturia. Diagnosis is confirmed by radioimmunoassay of serum PTH, which is elevated and reflects autonomous secretion.

Pathologically, the three main etiologies include adenoma, which is almost always limited to a single gland; hyperplasia, which affects all four glands; and carcinoma which, like adenoma, involves only one gland. Adenoma is the cause of primary hyperparathyroidism in nearly 80% of cases, hyperplasia in less than 20% of cases, and carcinoma in only 1%.

3.1.2 Secondary Hyperparathyroidism

Secondary hyperparathyroidism occurs as a reaction to a reduced total calcium pool and a low serum calcium level, the fluctuations of which modulate PTH secretion. Only secondary hyperparathyroidism linked to chronic renal failure is really important as it has then significant therapeutic implications. The other precipitating conditions (rickets, intestinal vitamin D malabsorption) are merely of physiopathological interest.

Certain signs observed during chronic renal failure are suggestive of secondary hyperparathyroidism: calcifications (arterial, corneal, conjunctival, periarticular, soft tissue), uremic pruritus refractory to hemodialysis and linked to subcutaneous calcium deposits, and bone pain (a rare sign of late onset).

Radiological studies classically demonstrate subperiosteal cortical bone erosion, "brown tumor" (local bone destruction), soft tissue calcification, and generalized deossification. Bone cysts are rare. Skeletal lesions are indicative of renal osteodystrophy, which regresses after parathyroidectomy.

3.1.3 Tertiary Hyperparathyroidism

Patients with chronic renal failure usually exhibit decreased or normal calcium concentrations, even when they suffer from severe hyperparathyroidism. Hypercalcemia can develop despite treatment aimed at lowering the hyperphosphatemia in patients undergoing hemodialysis and in renal transplant recipients as a result of autonomous parathyroid hyperfunction. Tertiary hyperparathyroidism is a rare pathology.

3.2 Histopathological Causes of Hyperparathyroidism

3.2.1 Parathyroid Adenoma

The location of an adenoma depends on the position of the normal parathyroid gland (cf. Chap. 1). The superior parathyroid gland (parathyroid IV) develops in association with the ultimobranchial or postbranchial body that participates in the formation of the lateral lobe of the thyroid gland. When discretely embedded in the capsule of the thyroid gland, a parathyroid gland may appear to be intrathyroidal. Multiple thyroid nodules can cause similar confusion, but true intrathyroid adenomas are extremely rare.

An adenoma located in the anterior mediastinum is the result of failure of the inferior parathyroid gland (parathyroid III) to separate from the thymus as the latter migrates downward; mediastinal adenomas occur in approximately 3% of patients and require thoracic surgery for ablation. Adenoma can also develop from a supernumerary parathyroid gland in the neck or mediastinum. Intrathyroidal, mediastinal, and supernumerary gland sites are all rare, and most adenomas involve the inferior parathyroid glands (parathyroid III).

On gross examination, adenomas are soft, encapsulated, reddish-brown masses; the surface may be lobulated and contain adipose or thymic tissue. The reddish-brown color of adenomas differs from both the hue of the thyroid and the opalescent gray of lymph nodes. Their shape varies with size: small adenomas tend to have the same ellipsoidal form as the parathyroid gland, whereas larger lesions may be spherical, oval, or bean-shaped. Calcifications are rare, but small cysts (1–10 mm) are fairly common. Cystic degeneration of parathyroid adenomas is rare and may be mistaken for a thyroid cyst.

3.2.2 Hyperplasia

The clinical picture of *chief-cell hyperplasia,* the most frequent type, is similar to that of adenoma except that the bone lesions are less extensive. One-fifth of cases are associated with a multiple endocrine neoplasia (MEN) syndrome (Castleman and Roth 1977). In MEN type I, hyperplasia of the parathyroid glands is associated with pancreatic islet tumors and pituitary adenomas; in MEN type II parathyroid hyperplasia, medullary thyroid cancer, and pheochromocytoma are associated (cf. Chap. 2).

On gross examination the lesions in parathyroid hyperplasia can vary in color from tan to reddish-brown and may contain small or large cysts. Of prime importance for diagnosis by imaging techniques is the fact that they are smaller than adenomas, often weighing only 1 g, and cannot be visualized by current imaging techniques. According to Castleman and Roth (1977), 50% of patients present with uniform hypertrophy of all the parathyroid glands; in the other 50%, only one of the glands is markedly enlarged; the other three are normal or only moderately enlarged.

Clear-cell hyperplasia, although defined as an entity before chief-cell hyperplasia, appears to be less common. Clear-cell hyperplasia has no distinguishing clinical features, but gross examination may reveal the absence of nodularity; lesions tend to be irregularly shaped and multilobular. For Castleman and Roth (1977) the superior parathyroid glands are often larger than the inferior glands, which may even be smaller than normal.

3.2.3 Parathyroid Carcinoma

The most common cause of parathyroid cancer is a functioning adenocarcinoma, which can be the cause of fatal hypercalcemia (Murie et al. 1973). Parathyroid carcinoma accounts for approximately 1% of all cases of primary hyperparathyroidism, and affects males and females in equal numbers, as opposed to benign tumors.

The clinical course may correspond to either a critical situation from the outset, with acute hyperparathyroidism but no concomitant renal or bone lesions, or a chronic condition subject to slow or rapid deterioration. Presenting signs usually include asthenia, weight loss, and a combination of psychoneurologic, gastrointestinal, and renal symptoms reflecting the severity of hypercalcemia (generally over 140 mg/liter). Parathyroid hormone levels are also elevated. Of particular interest is the fact that nearly 70% of parathyroid cancers are palpable, whereas adenomas and hyperplasia generally are not. Postoperative recurrence of hyperparathyroidism after surgical excision of what was presumed to be an adenoma should also suggest malignancy (Holmes et al. 1969). Both intraoperative identification and postoperative diagnosis of parathyroid carcinoma remain extremely difficult; the only reliable criteria of malignancy are nodal metastases and the invasion of adjacent structures. The presence of neoplastic vascular emboli is also helpful for diagnosis, but nuclear anomalies cannot be relied on as they also occur in adenomas. Intraoperative diagnosis is only possible in cases of patent spread to surrounding tissue or metastasis to lymph nodes.

Visceral metastases are rare, but postoperative disease recurrence is fairly common (30%-60% of cases), even after apparently successful surgical excision. The prognosis for parathyroid carcinoma is less than 25% at 10 years (Castleman and Roth 1977).

3.2.4 Other Histologic Forms

Two additional pathologies also warrant mention. *Nonfunctioning lesions* are exceedingly rare, but merit consideration because they can easily be confused clinically, and occasionally even on imaging studies, with a thyroid tumor. Accurate localization of nonfunctioning adenomas, cysts, and, more rarely, undifferentiated carcinoma generally requires surgery or histological examination; a thyroid pathology is usually the prospective diagnostic consideration prior to surgery.

Tumor-related hypercalcemia can prove difficult to differentiate from primary hyperparathyroidism. Even today, a formal diagnosis may remain impossible if a thorough workup fails to detect malignancy, especially since 60% of patients with tumor-related hypercalcemia have lung or renal carcinoma also. Biochemical tests are not always conclusive, but classical signs suggestive of tumor-related hypercalcemia include sudden onset, the absence of bone or urinary lesions, and a discrepancy between a very high calcium concentration and a moderate parathyroid hormone level.

3.3 Ultrasonography

To be efficient, diagnostic ultrasound requires the examiner to be familiar with the normal anatomic distribution of the parathyroid glands as well as with the possible variations in their location and number (Moreau and Carlier-Conrads 1984) (cf. Chap. 1).

3.3.1 Ultrasonographic Features of Primary Hyperparathyroidism

Regardless of their etiology (adenoma, hyperplasia, cancer) parathyroid masses are hypoechogenic or anechoic; their internal architecture is usually homogeneous. Lesions with a cystic component (multiple, small cysts are more common than a single, large area) are characteristically inhomogeneous. Calcifications are rare (Figs. 3.1; 3.10). The sonographic pattern cannot be used to differentiate between benign and malignant lesions. By contrast, nonmobile lesions (expecially those fixed to deep structures) and concomitant nodal masses are suggestive of a neoplastic process. The shape of single or multiple lesions usually depends on their location:

- retrothyroid lesions tend to be oval or very flat, and are separated from the thyroid by a clearly defined line; the presence of a halo is rare
- infrathyroid nodules are generally spherical owing to elongation of their anteroposterior diameter

Regardless of their position, and except for those rare tumors which are obviously cancerous because neighboring tissue is invaded, parathyroid lesions are mobile when the patient swallows, and move along with the thyroid gland. Real-time examination shows such nodules moving up and down along the longus colli muscle, which itself remains stationary. Ultrasonography can also visualize parathyroid cysts (DeRaimo et al. 1984; Krudy et al. 1984c) and multiple lesions (multiple adenomas or hyperplasia characterized by unusually large glands) (Manhire et al. 1984).

Familiarity with the most frequent sites of ectopic glands (submaxillary region, within the thyroid, at the cervicothoracic junction) is essential for thorough US examination. Intrathyroid parathyroid adenomas occur in 1%-2% of cases, and although these nodules have no specific ultrasonic characteristics, there is usually a clearly defined separation between the nodule and the adjacent thyroid parenchyma. As thyroid lesions are frequently associated with hyperparathyroidism, and in view of the possibility of an intrathyroidal parathyroid adenoma, the sonographer should be particularly meticu-

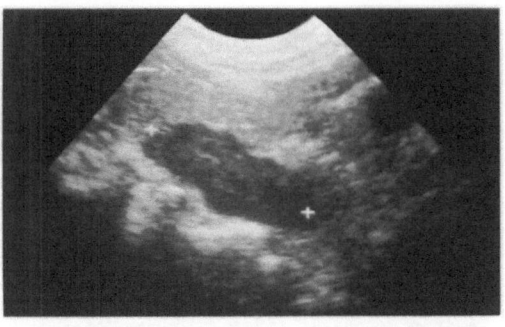

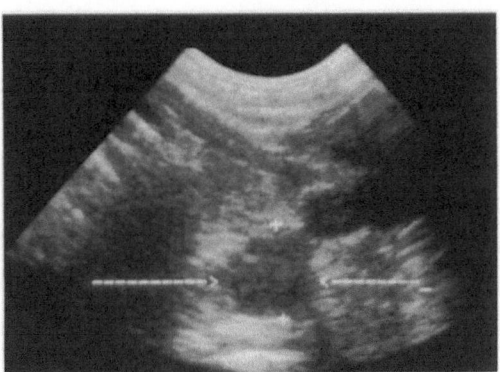

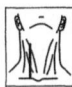 **Fig. 3.1.** Parathyroid adenoma of decreased echogenicity relative to the adjacent thyroid tissue (sagittal scan) (27 mm between the two *crosses*)

 Fig. 3.2. Small (8 mm) adenoma *(arrows)* much more echogenic than the surrounding thyroid parenchyma (transverse scan)

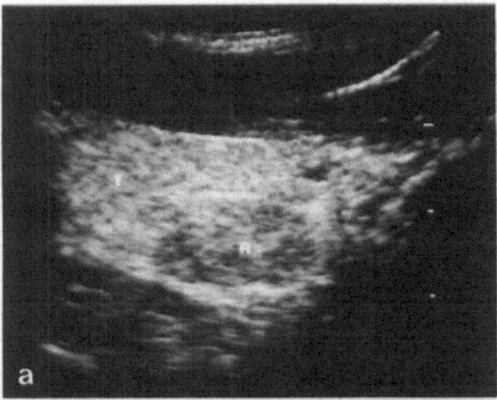

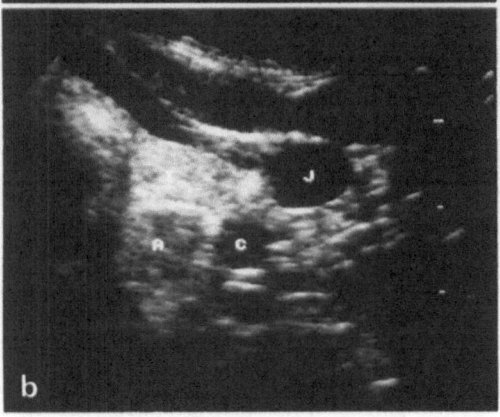

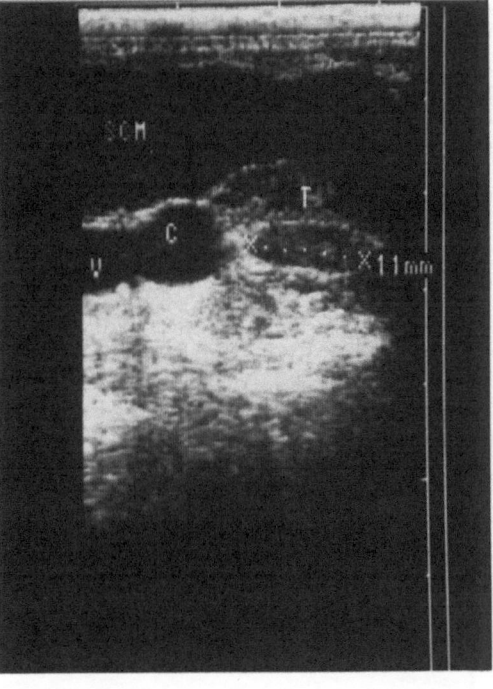

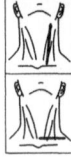 **Fig. 3.3 a, b.** Sagittal (a) and transverse (b) scans of a parathyroid adenoma *(A)* that is strongly hypoechogenic relative to the thyroid *(T)*. The cervical vessels can be seen laterally on the transverse scan. *C,* common carotid artery; *J,* jugular vein

 Fig. 3.4. Adenoma of the right retrothyroid upper parathyroid gland (parathyroid IV) (transverse scan) (11 mm between the two *crosses*). *SCM,* sternocleidomastoid muscle; *T,* thyroid gland; *C,* common carotid artery; *V,* jugular vein

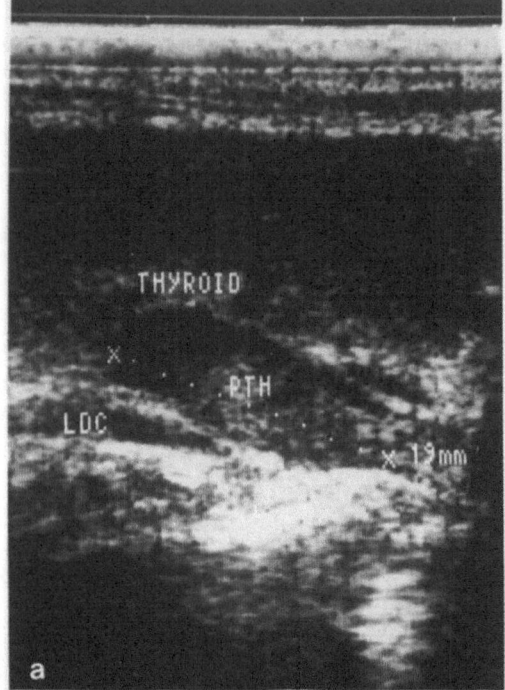

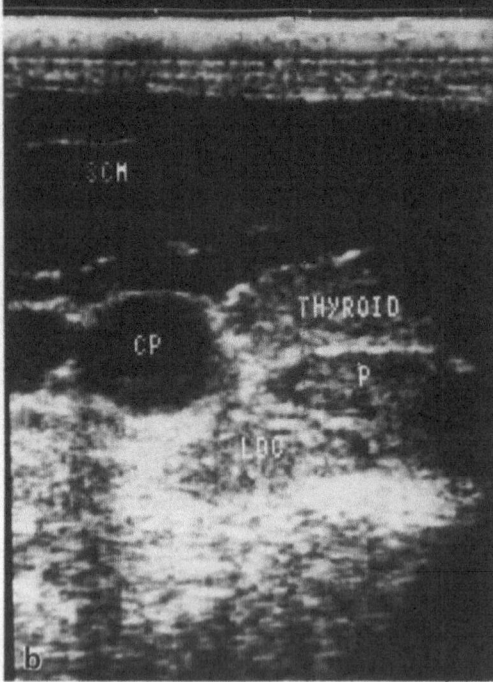

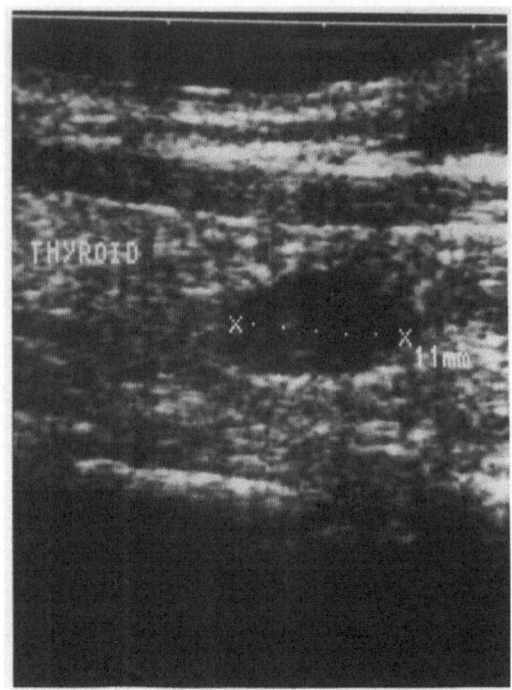

Fig. 3.6. Left parathyroid III adenoma slightly below the lower pole of the thyroid lobe (sagittal scan) (11 mm between the two *crosses*)

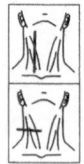

Fig. 3.5 a, b. Sagittal (**a**) and transverse (**b**) scans of a parathyroid adenoma (19 mm between the two *crosses*) in a partly retrotracheal upper right location. *CP*, common carotid artery; *SCM*, sternocleidomastoid muscle; *LDC*, longus colli muscle; *PTH* and *P*, parathyroid adenoma

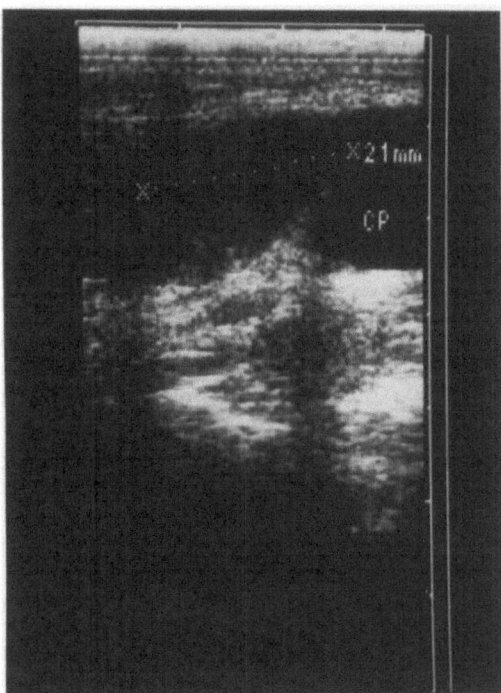

 Fig. 3.7. Parathyroid III adenoma located entirely within the infrathyroid space (21 mm between the two *crosses*); no thyroid covering (transverse scan). *CP*, common carotid artery

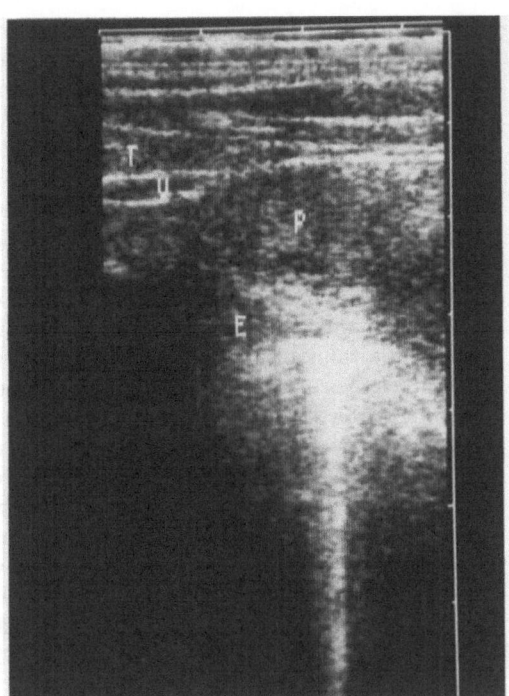

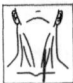 **Fig. 3.8.** Left cervicomediastinal parathyroid adenoma; the lower portion is hidden by the clavicle (sagittal scan). *T,* lower part of the left thyroid lobe; *V,* inferior thyroid vein; *E,* esophagus; *P,* parathyroid adenoma

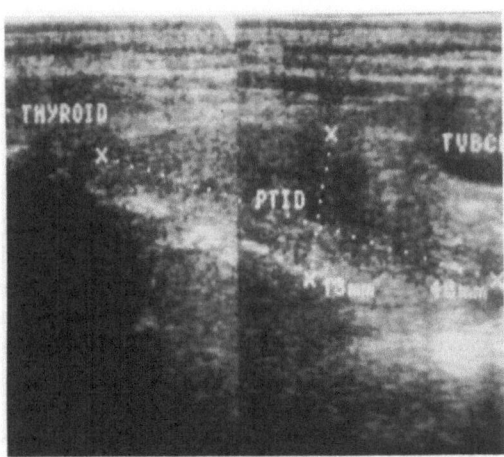

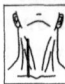 **Fig. 3.9.** Large parathyroid IV adenoma (18 mm × 48 mm) occupying the entire infrathyroid space in a tall, thin individual (sagittal scan). *TVBC,* right innominate vein; *PTID,* right parathyroid adenoma

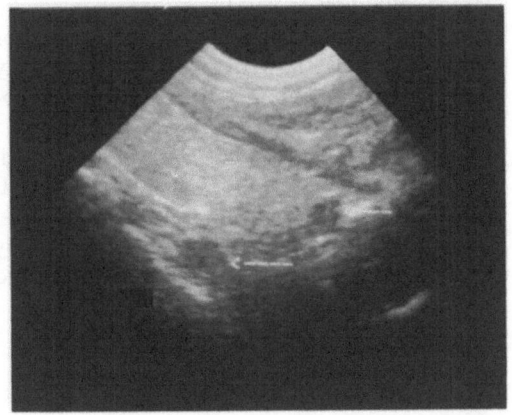

 Fig. 3.10. Two hyperplastic right parathyroid lesions *(arrows)* (sagittal scan)

lous in indicating the existence and locations of any thyroid nodules even in a clinical setting of hyperthyroidism. Infrathyroid superior parathyroid glands (parathyroid IV) account for most cases of ectopia (5%–10%); they lie deep to the vertebrae, often in a cervicomediastinal location. Retroesophageal and mediastinal masses are totally inaccessible to ultrasound, but they represent less than 10% of cases.

Ever since the results published by Sample et al. (1978), numerous publications have demonstrated the value of ultrasonography for parathyroid studies. Analysis of 200 literature cases reported from 1984 to 1986 credits US with a sensitivity of 66%–84% and a diagnostic accuracy of 87%–94%. In addition to the improvements brought about in examination quality by real-time equipment and high-frequency transducers, the expertise of the sonographer plays an important role in the diagnosis of hyperparathyroidism (Moreau et al. 1980; Reading et al. 1982; Sample et al. 1978; Simeone et al. 1981; Stark et al. 1983a).

3.3.2 Ultrasonographic Features of Secondary Hyperparathyroidism

The parathyroid glands of patients with advanced hyperparathyroidism are usually all enlarged, although to varying degrees; in severe cases, the largest glands may weigh up to 4 or 5 g. The glands show decreased echogenicity and tend to be more spherical than adenomas.

Systematic US investigation of patients with chronic renal failure appears justified, especially for those requiring long-term hemodialysis. Comparison of serial sonograms permits easy detection and precise localization of any rapid increase in gland size.

3.3.3 False-Negative Ultrasonography

Patient-related sources of false-negative errors include poor quality examinations resulting from the patient's inability to keep his neck hyperextended; this problem is common in elderly patients with cervical arthrosis or vascular problems, or who experience dyspnea when supine. Cutaneous atrophy and sclerosis of the

infrahyoid muscles in older patients can also render examination difficult; the same is true for scar tissue. Because young children may find the examination hard to tolerate, there is a risk that thorough studies will not be obtained.

False-negative errors attributed to the inexperience of the operator may actually be due to problems inherent in parathyroid studies:

– small size is not the only reason why adenomas escape detection, at least for lesions up to 5 mm in diameter; most errors occur when the parathyroid mass lies outside the thyroid capsule or when the thyroid tissue is itself diseased. It should be kept in mind that only the superior parathyroid glands are covered by the thyroid gland; most inferior parathyroid glands are only slightly or not at all covered by thyroid parenchyma.

– as infrathyroid lesions account for the majority of false-negative errors, thorough exploration of the lower neck is essential.

– whether they have an extensive cystic component or are associated with thyroid nodules, the parathyroid origin of certain large adenomas may escape detection if only lesions less than 2 cm in greatest dimension are expected.

3.3.4 False-Positive Ultrasonography

False-positive errors are a much greater problem for the surgeon than false-negatives. Certain false-positives result from lack of familiarity with the normal anatomy of the neck, especially the blood vessels and longus colli muscle. When the esophagus deviates laterally into the left side of the neck, it can nearly always be seen from the thyroid isthmus to the clavicle. The bull's-eye appearance of a lateralized esophagus may be modified on transverse scans with alteration of the central US pattern (the central hyperechogenic image may be replaced by a slightly fluidlike or hypoechogenic zone when the patient swallows saliva on request). Real-time examination can prevent interpretive errors.

Pathological vascular structures, such as atheromatous and winding carotid arteries, can also be a source of error. In elderly patients unable to keep their neck hyperextended, even the use of a real-time transducer does not always allow differentiation of a vessel from a possible parathyroid pathology. Confusion of a parathyroid lesion with an enlarged node is less common, as adenopathies are generally located more laterally in the neck; small adenopathies are usually closely applied to the carotid artery and the internal jugular vein. Confusion with a node of the recurrent nerve chain is also theoretically possible, but no such errors have been reported in the literature.

The major cause of false-positive error is a symptomatic thyroid nodule, encountered in 20% of patients with hyperparathyroidism (Moreau and Carlier-Conrads 1984). Localization of hyperechogenic nodules is not difficult as there are no hyperechogenic parathyroid tumors, but a peripherally situated hypoechogenic nodule can involve serious diagnostic problems.

3.3.5 Diagnostic and Therapeutic Aspiration Biopsy Under Ultrasonographic Guidance

Solbiati et al. (1983) have reported using fine-needle biopsy under ultrasonographic guidance for both primary and secondary hyperparathyroidism with a sensitivity of 81.5% and a diagnostic accuracy of 86.5%. In addition to the information provided by histological examination, radioimmunoassay allows measurement of parathyroid hormone in the biopsy material (Krudy et al. 1984a) (Fig. 3.11).

Along with biopsies for diagnostic purposes, percutaneous injection of absolute ethanol into parathyroid lesions under ultrasonographic guidance has been proposed as a therapeutic procedure (Solbiati et al. 1985). Alcoholic ablation is essentially reserved for patients with secondary hyperparathyroidism, when only one gland is hyperplastic, or when the patient is in poor clinical condition or refuses surgery. In their treatment protocol, Solbiati et al. (1985) injected tumors with 1–2.5 cc of ethanol under US guidance; significant reductions in lesion size were observed over the next 6 months in 75% of cases. Structural changes resulting from alcoholic ablation included the appearance of hyperechogenic images secondary to fibrosis and a few rare instances of anechoic masses

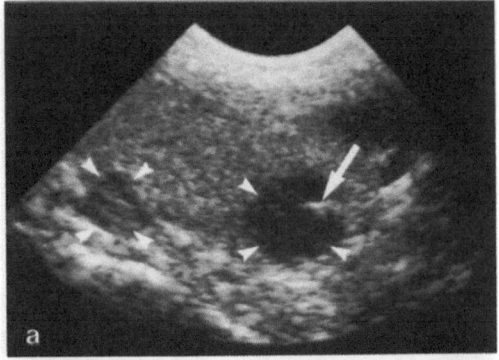

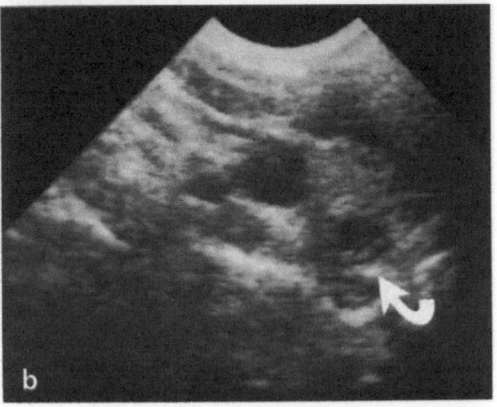

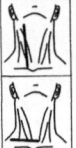

Fig. 3.11 a, b. Aspiration biopsy of a parathyroid adenoma (**a** sagittal scan): visualization of two parathyroid tumors *(small arrows)*; the bright echo corresponds to the tip of the needle *(large arrow)* in the lower tumor during aspiration. In **b** (oblique scan) the distal portion of the needle is visible *(arrow)*. Courtesy of Dr. Solbiati

corresponding to necrosis. The habitual absence of complications with this procedure makes it a useful technique, at least for patients with secondary hyperparathyroidism.

3.3.6 Intraoperative Ultrasonography

The basic purpose of this little utilized procedure is shortening of the operative time required for lesion localization. Intraoperative exploration is not possible for the entire cervical region, however, and the posterior regions are particularly hard to scan, as emphasized by Sigel et al. (1981) (Figs. 3.12 and 3.13).

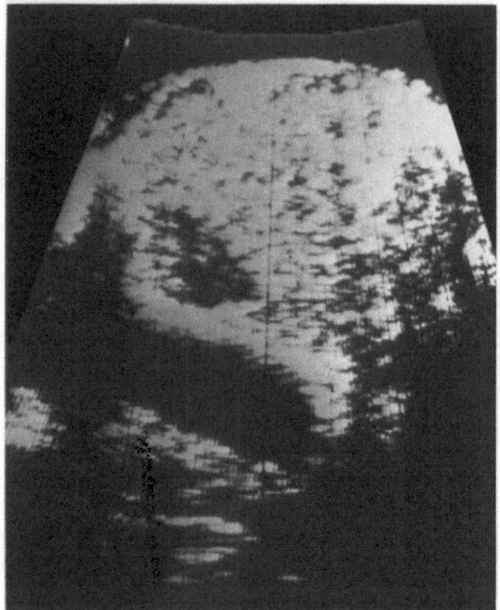

Fig. 3.12. Intraoperative ultrasonography of the lateral neck showing a small parathyroid adenoma near the common carotid artery. Courtesy of Dr. Hernigou and Professor Plainfossé

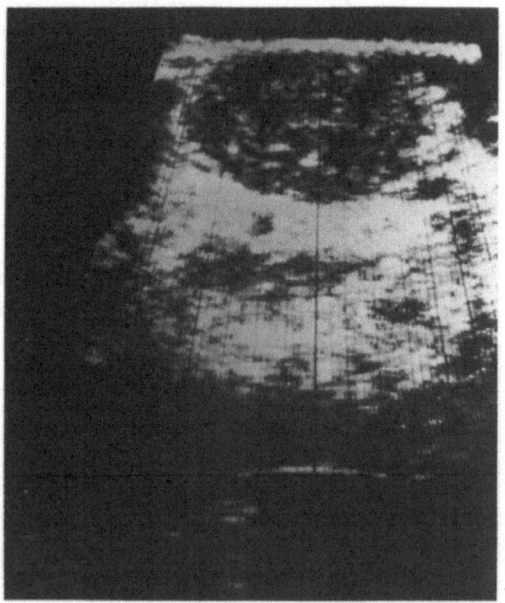

Fig. 3.13. Intraoperative ultrasonography of the lateral neck: large, palpable parathyroid adenomas anterior to a small, nonpalpable hyperplastic parathyroid gland. Courtesy of Dr. Hernigou and Professor Plainfossé

3.4 Nonultrasonographic Techniques

The major nonultrasonographic procedures for parathyroid gland investigations include: barium swallow, radioisotope scanning with thallium, computed tomography, arteriography, and venous sampling.

3.4.1 Barium Swallow (Esophagram)

Both the sensitivity and the specificity (false-positives due to thyroid disease) of this classical technique are low. Despite this, as an accurate examination of the retrotracheal and retroesophageal regions is difficult with US, a barium swallow can often reveal adenomas in these sites. Barium swallows are no longer the preferred diagnostic procedure for parathyroid lesions, but they remain useful for posterior sites if sonograms are noncontributory.

3.4.2 Radioisotope Scanning

Radioisotope scanning of the parathyroid glands is currently performed with thallium-201; as this radionuclide is concentrated by the thyroid as well as by the parathyroid glands, the thyroid image is subtracted following marking with another isotope (technetium-99m or iodine-123). Certain authors credit this technique with a sensitivity of up to 90% (Corcoran et al. 1983) and have reported success in detecting lesions as small as 5 mm in diameter.

3.4.3 Computed Tomography (CT)

When performed with rapid scan times and contrast material in a patient who can maintain sufficient hyperextension providing access to almost the entire cervicothoracic region, CT is superior to ultrasonography. The retrotracheal-retroesophageal region inaccessible to US is well analyzed by CT, and mediastinal investigations are also satisfactory (the posterior mediastinum is involved less often than the anterior mediastinum) (Doppman et al. 1982). Overall, CT is 5%–10% more sensitive than ultrasound.

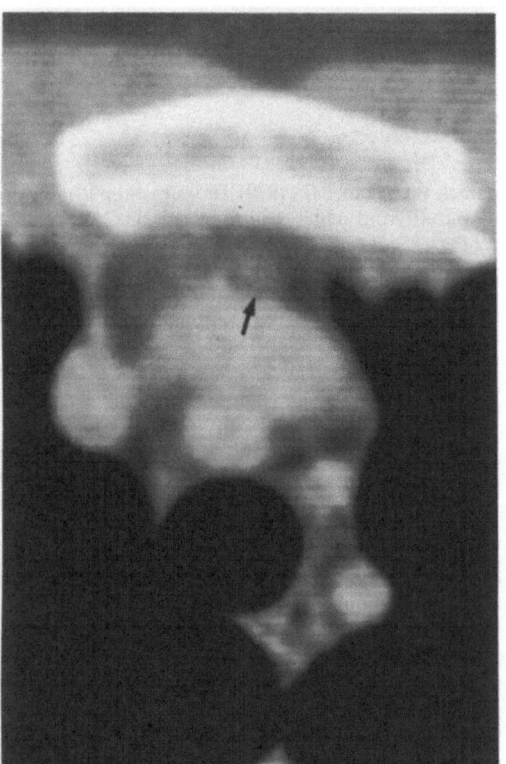

Fig. 3.14. CT scan of the upper mediastinum showing a small parathyroid adenoma misdiagnosed by US *(arrow)*. Courtesy of Dr. Drouillard

Despite its many advantages, CT has several technical limitations: lesion size (lesions under 5 mm in diameter cannot be visualized), motion artifacts caused by respiration and swallowing, and interference from metal surgical clips or fibrosis following an initial cervical exploration. Diagnostic confusions encountered with CT include the possible vertical orientation of a gland in the neck, the possibility of asymmetry of the thyroid lobes or other cervical structures, and cervical adenopathies. Other problems are the frequency of associated thyroid lesions, imaging difficulties due to a sparsity of cervical or mediastinal fat, and the tortuous nature of certain vessels (Drouillard et al. 1983; Sommer et al. 1982; Stark et al. 1983b; Tagaki et al. 1982) (Fig. 3.14).

3.4.4 Arteriography

Arteriography of a parathyroid mass requires selective injection of contrast material into the inferior thyroid artery, the internal mammary artery, and the superior thyroid artery. Adenomas in the anterior mediastinum are usually supplied by a descending branch of the inferior thyroid artery or a thymic branch of the internal mammary artery. Both adenomas and carcinomas are usually hypervascularized (Krudy et al. 1981, 1982).

Mediastinal lesions can be treated by embolization or infusion of contrast material through a wedged catheter (Doppman et al. 1981). These procedures are restricted to patients who have already had an unsuccessful neck exploration. Embolization can obviate the need for reoperation if it succeeds in bringing calcium and parathyroid hormone levels back to normal.

Digital subtraction angiography (DSA) remains of questionable value. Venous DSA has been judged unsuitable for screening purposes (Obley et al. 1984), and the sensitivity of arterial DSA with injection into the aorta is reportedly insufficient for mediastinal lesions (Krudy et al. 1984b). At present, selective catheterization still appears necessary for localization of mediastinal disease sites.

3.4.5 Venous Sampling

Venography is required before venous sampling can be performed as variations exist in the number and drainage of vessels. After delineation of the vascular anatomy, samples are taken from the thyroid veins (in particular the inferior thyroid veins), the jugular veins, and the innominate trunks. Care must also be taken to evaluate thymic drainage. Sample points are recorded on a chart, and parathyroid hormone measurements must be interpreted with reference to the venogram.

Thorough venous sampling is not always possible, especially when previous surgery has altered venous drainage (ligation or venous thrombosis). Despite a diagnostic accuracy of less than 75%, venous sampling is indicated after a failed initial neck exploration and when neither CT nor internal mammary arteriography succeed in localizing an ectopic adenoma (Krudy et al. 1981).

3.5 Role of Ultrasonography in the Imaging of Hyperparathyroidism

For patients with secondary hyperparathyroidism, ultrasonography is often the only examination required; alcoholic ablation of nodules under ultrasonic guidance can be a valid alternative to surgery. The most controversial yet potentially most valuable use of ultrasonography concerns primary hyperparathyroidism. Although neck exploration remains mandatory for hypercalcemic patients with an elevated parathyroid hormone level, ultrasonography is an inexpensive, noninvasive, and quite sensitive means of assessing future surgical difficulties. Preoperative ultrasound localization of a parathyroid lesion can be a great aid for the surgeon. Likewise, a negative study obtained by an experienced sonographer should orient the search toward a posterior cervical site or raise the possibility of multigland hyperplasia rather than adenoma. CT should be performed for patients with primary hyperparathyroidism who have normal ultrasound studies.

Imaging techniques in general, and ultrasonography in particular, have unquestionably benefited the workup of patients with hyperparathyroidism. They are aids for the selection of the best surgical procedure rather than determinants of the therapeutic approach, as surgery is the only means of obtaining a cure. Despite its utilization for both diagnostic and therapeutic purposes in secondary hyperparathyroidism, US of patients with primary hyperparathyroidism remains solely a diagnostic procedure. It thus seems legitimate to suggest cervical ultrasonography as the initial examination; if lesions are visualized, no other examinations are required. Mediastinal CT is not indispensable. Owing to the generally satisfactory sensitivity of US, a normal sonogram should suggest the possibility of an ectopic gland, in which case CT is advisable. If surgical neck exploration fails to discover the cause of hyperparathyroidism, a search must be made before reoperation for an ectopic hypertrophic gland or a gland that has escaped surgical detection, first by US, then by CT. These can be followed, if necessary, by arteriography, in particular to search for a mediastinal lesion that may be amenable to embolization, and venous sampling. As venous sampling can be difficult in patients with surgical antecedents, it should remain the technique of last resort.

3.6 References

Black WC, Haff RC (1970) The surgical pathology of parathyroid chief cell hyperplasia. Am J Clin Path 53: 565–571

Boonstra CE, Jackson CE (1965) Hyperparathyroidism detected by routine serum calcium analysis. Prevalence in a clinic population. Ann Intern Med 63: 468–479

Castleman B, Roth SI (1977) Tumors of the parathyroid glands. Atlas of tumor pathology, 2nd series, Fasc 14. AFIP, Washington DC

Corcoran MO, Seifacian MA, George SL, Milroy E (1983) Location of parathyroid adenomas by thallium 201 and technetium 99m subtraction scanning. Br Med J 286: 1751–1752

De Raimo AJ, Kane RA, Katz JF, Rolla AP (1984) Parathyroid cyst: diagnosis by sonography and needle aspiration. AJR 142: 1227–1228

Doppman JL, Popovsky M, Girton M (1981) The use of iodinated contrast agents to ablate organs; experimental studies and histopathology. Radiology 138: 333–340

Doppman JL, Krudy AG, Brennan MF, Schneider P, Lasker RD, Marx SJ (1982) CT appearance of enlarged parathyroid glands in the posterior superior mediastinum. J Comput Assist Tomogr 6: 1099–1102

Drouillard J, Philippe JC, Erésué J, Rollet JC, Roux P, Pastaud P, Guichard F, Tavernier J (1983) Place de la scanographie dans le diagnostic des adénomes parathyroïdiens. A propos de 27 cas. J Radiol 64: 381–390

Holmes EC, Morton DL, Ketcham AS (1969) Parathyroid carcinoma: a collective review. Ann Surg 169: 631–640

Krudy AG, Doppman JL, Brennan MF, Marx SJ, Spiegel AM, Stock JL, Aurbach GD (1981) The detection of mediastinal parathyroid glands by computed tomography, selective angiography and venous sampling. An analysis of 17 cases. Radiology 140: 739–744

Krudy AG, Doppman JL, Marx SJ, Brennan MF, Spiegel A, Aurbach GD (1982) Radiographic findings in recurrent parathyroid carcinoma. Radiology 142: 625–629

Krudy AG, Doppman JL, Marx SJ, Norton JA, Spiegel AM, Santora AC II, Aurbach GD (1984a) Parathyroid aspiration directed by angiography: an alternative to venous sampling. Radiology 152: 207–208

Krudy AG, Doppman JL, Miller DL, Norton JA, Marx SJ, Spiegel AM, Santora AC II, Aurbach GD, Schaaf M (1984b) Detection of mediastinal parathyroid glands by nonselective digital arteriography. AJR 142: 693–695

Krudy AG, Doppman JL, Shawker TH, Spiegel AM, Marx SJ, Norton J, Schaaf M, Moss ML, Weiss MA, Schachner SH (1984c) Hyperfunctioning cystic parathyroid glands: CT and sonographic findings. AJR 142: 175–178

Manhire AR, Anderson PN, Milroy E (1984) Parathyroid venous sampling and ultrasonography in primary parathyroidism due to multigland disease. Br J Radiol 57: 375–380

Moreau JF, Carlier-Conrads L (1984) Imagerie diagnostique des glandes thyroïde et parathyroïdes. Vigot, Paris

Moreau JF, Ulmann A, Drueke T, Hamidou S, Dubost C (1980) Localization of parathyroid tumors by ultrasonography. N Engl J Med 302: 582–583

Murie N, Ferrand D, Etienne P (1973) Le cancer des parathyroïdes. Revue générale de 109 observations. Nouv Presse Med 2: 1293–1296

Obley DL, Winzelberg GG, Jarmolowski CR, Hydovitz JD, Danowski TS, Wholey MH (1984) Parathyroid adenomas studied by digital subtraction angiography. Radiology 153: 449–451

Reading CC, Charboneau JW, James EM, Karsell PR, Purnell DC, Grant CS, Van Heerden JA (1982) High-resolution parathyroid sonography. AJR 139: 539–546

Sample WF, Mitchell SP, Bledsoe RC (1978) Parathyroid ultrasonography. Radiology 127: 485–490

Sigel B, Kraft AR, Nyhus LM, Coelho JCU, Favin MP, Spigos DG (1981) Identification of a parathyroid adenoma by operative ultrasound. Arch Surg 116: 234–235

Simeone JF, Mueller PR, Ferrucci JT Jr, Van Sonnenberg E, Wang CA, Hall DA, Wittenberg J (1981) High-resolution real-time sonography of the parathyroid. Radiology 141: 745–751

Solbiati L, Montali G, Croce F, Bellotti E, Giangrande A, Ravetto C (1983) Parathyroid tumors detected by fine-needle aspiration biopsy under ultrasonic guidance. Radiology 148: 793–797

Solbiati L, Giangrande A, Ierace T, Rizatto G, Derchi LE (1985) Treatment of parathyroid tumors in secondary hyperparathyroidism by percutaneous ethanol injection under ultrasonic guidance. J Ultrasound Med 4: 12

Sommer B, Welter HF, Spelsberg F, Scherer U, Lissner J (1982) Computed tomography for localizing enlarged parathyroid glands in primary hyperparathyroidism. J Comput Assist Tomogr 6: 521–526

Stark DD, Gooding GAW, Moss AA, Clark OH, Ovenfors CO (1983a) Parathyroid imaging: comparison of high-resolution CT and high-resolution sonography. AJR 141: 633–638

Stark DD, Moss AA, Gooding GAW, Clark OH (1983b) Parathyroid scanning by computed tomography. Radiology 148: 297–299

Takagi H, Tominaga Y, Uchida K, Yamada N, Ishii T, Morimoto T, Yasue M (1982) Preoperative diagnosis of secondary hyperparathyroidism using computed tomography. J Comput Assist Tomogr 6: 527–528

4 Salivary Glands

J.-N. Bruneton, F. Normand, N. Santini, and C. Balu-Maestro

The ultrasonographic appearance of the normal salivary glands has already been described in Chap. 1, so the present discussion will detail the nonultrasonographic techniques available for salivary gland studies and review the tumoral and infectious pathologies of these glands together with nontumoral, noninflammatory pathologies. The value of ultrasonography (US) is most evident in the workup of salivary gland tumors (Baker and Ossoinig 1977; Ballerini et al. 1984; Bruneton et al. 1980; Bruneton and Roux 1984). A limited number of other publications have reported ultrasonography to be effective in the analysis of inflammatory and lithiasic disorders (Bellina 1982; Hajek et al. 1984; Pickrell et al. 1978).

4.1 Nonultrasonographic Imaging Techniques

In the years to come, magnetic resonance imaging using surface coils will probably prove to be the most sensitive technique for the anatomic analysis of salivary gland tumors. Preliminary results are extremely promising, even though the limited size of series to date precludes global evaluation. The remainder of this section has therefore been restricted to sialography, computed tomography, and scintigraphy, the three main imaging procedures currently used for investigations of the salivary glands.

4.1.1 Sialography

Owing to the minimal amount of equipment required for sialography, the oldest radiological technique for salivary gland explorations, this examination can be performed almost anywhere. Although the usefulness of the method for tumoral pathologies has decreased since the introduction of US and CT, sialograms are particularly indicated in inflammatory disease because of their superior definition of anatomic detail.

Failed cannulation of the submandibular or parotid ducts seldom occurs when the procedure is performed by an experienced operator; such failures generally represent less than 10% of cases. Sialography is not performed until after plain films have been taken (anteroposterior, tangential, lateral, and axial views for the parotid gland; anteroposterior and a lateral oblique jaw view for the submandibular gland). Preinjection radiographs are followed by films taken during filling with contrast material and after evacuation. Tomographic, magnification, and subtraction techniques all increase the procedure's sensitivity. Sialography is highly accurate for analysis of intraductal lesions as well as for inflammatory and infectious diseases of the salivary glands.

The interest of using sialography for tumoral investigations is currently limited as less invasive but equally sensitive procedures are available; the average sensitivity of sialography is between 75% and 90% (Calcaterra et al. 1977; Einstein 1966; Gates 1971; Kushner and Weber 1978). Sialography can be combined with CT for the investigation of space-occupying lesions, and it remains indicated for differentiation of inflammatory disease from a tumor.

4.1.2 Computed Tomography

Contiguous 5-mm thick slices are obtained in the transverse projection, completed whenever possible by coronal scans (Bryan et al. 1982; Eyjolfsson et al. 1984; McGahan et al. 1984; Mancuso and Hanafee 1982; Som and Biller 1980). As dental amalgams can create artifacts on CT scans, the position of the patient's neck may have to be modified for coronal or transverse scanning.

Parotid gland explorations must be completed by an examination of the neck because tumoral processes can be accompanied by nodal involvement. Owing to the vascular relations of the parotid, an intravenous contrast material must be utilized for thorough evaluation.

The CT density of the normal parotid gland is between -30 and -10 HU, in other words between that of the fat in the adjacent tissue and that of the surrounding muscles. Except when hindered by dental artifacts, CT can accurately analyze the deep parotid lobe; it is particularly useful for demonstrating tumoral spread from the deep lobe and lesions arising in the parapharyngeal space. Not all authors agree on the utility of systematically coupling sialography with CT, especially when a high-resolution CT scanner is available. In theory CT sialography allows analysis of the facial nerve as it courses through the parotid gland; however, the data obtained corresponds to anatomic predictions because CT, like US, cannot actually visualize the facial nerve. According to Conn et al. (1983) "the nerve could be represented on a CT scan by an arc of radius 8.5 mm, the centre of which is the most posterior point of the ramus of the mandible."

The primary indication for CT is the evaluation of tumoral pathologies: even though lithiasis can be analyzed by CT, inflammatory disorders are best studied by sialography. CT of the submandibular gland also seems limited to the workup of tumors; however, good quality coronal scans are easier to obtain here as the submandibular gland is located anteriorly relative to the parotid gland.

4.1.3 Scintigraphy

Salivary scintigraphy is a noninvasive procedure that relies on the intravenous injection of ^{99m}Tc sodium pertechnetate. Along with dynamic flow studies, static images can be obtained in the Waters, right lateral, and left lateral positions. Analysis of obstructive disease requires delayed films 24 h after injection.

The basic purpose of scintigraphy is evaluation of the functional status of the salivary glands; the major and minor salivary glands are nor-

mally visualized together as anatomically and functionally symmetrical structures. For patients with sialolithiasis, scintiscans are a helpful means of assessing gland function prior to surgery. The various situations ranging from normal to complete nonfunction are conditioned by the extent of any ductal obstruction or complications.

By contrast, scintigraphy has no specificity for tumors. Salivary gland tumors generally present as "cold" filling defects, although "hot" lesions of increased activity are possible. This is namely the case with cystadenolymphoma and certain cancers such as mucoepidermoid carcinoma. The "warm" activity of such tumors reflects the concentration of ^{99m}Tc pertechnetate due to the tumor's salivary ductal epithelium origin (Ohrt and Shafer 1982).

The principal application of scintigraphy is the workup of patients with Sjögren's syndrome, a disease characterized by a diffuse decrease in the uptake of all of the salivary glands; the efficacy of therapy for Sjögren's syndrome can also be evaluated from scintiscans (Schmitt et al. 1976).

4.2 Tumors of the Salivary Glands

In their review Thackray and Lucas (1974) estimated the incidence of salivary gland tumors at less than 3 per 100000 population. Certain geographic variations have been reported, however, and Eskimos, for some still unexplained reason, show a high prevalence of such tumors.

Tumors are 10 to 15 times more common in the parotid gland than in the submandibular glands (Eneroth 1971; Thackray and Lucas 1974). Benign lesions, essentially adenomas, account for 85%-90% of all parotid tumors. Except when presenting symptoms are suggestive of malignancy (large rapidly growing tumor, facial paralysis, nodal masses), 9 out of 10 parotid tumors are thus benign. By contrast, all submandibular tumors should be considered highly suspicious owing to the frequency of cancers of this anatomic site (33%), even after the possibility of metastatic nodes of lingual cancer has been ruled out.

4.2.1 Benign Salivary Gland Tumors

4.2.1.1 Pleomorphic Adenoma

Pleomorphic adenoma, or mixed tumor, is the most frequent (60%–70%) tumoral lesion of the salivary glands. This slow-growing tumor is composed of epithelial cells and varying proportions of mucoid, chondroid, and myxoid tissue. Pleomorphic adenoma is nearly 10 times more common in the parotid gland than in the submandibular gland. Women tend to be affected more often than men, and patients are usually 40 years old or more at diagnosis. Approximately 90% of mixed tumors of the parotid occur in the superficial lobe (Thackray and Lucas 1974), thus ultrasonography is particularly indicated for imaging studies.

The gross appearance of a pleomorphic adenoma is a solid mass with a bosselated surface. Hemorrhagic or cystic degeneration of surface protuberances (lobed processes) may be present. Above all, at least 25% of all mixed tumors are associated with satellite nodules separate from the main tumor; such findings have fueled debate as to the possibility of a multicentric origin. Owing to the propensity of pleomorphic adenoma to recur locally after surgical excision by enucleation, total parotidectomy is warranted. The possibility of *malignant transformation* of a pleomorphic adenoma remains controversial and has yet to be proven conclusively; even so, the appearance of certain highly differentiated histological forms of cancer closely resembles that of pleomorphic adenoma.

Sonographically, pleomorphic adenoma habitually presents all of the features of benignity when its greatest dimension is less than 3 cm. Well-circumscribed parotid lesions with a homogeneous ultrasonic pattern can be considered benign. The absence of either sharp margins or internal homogenity on sonograms suggests malignancy. A pleomorphic adenoma smaller than 3 cm is usually visualized as a nodule of decreased echogenicity relative to the remainder of the gland; the ultrasonic pattern is homogeneous and the margins are well delimited (Bruneton et al. 1980; Neiman et al. 1976). Discrete posterior reinforcement may be visible, especially if the nodule is strongly hypoechogenic (Figs. 4.1–4.8).

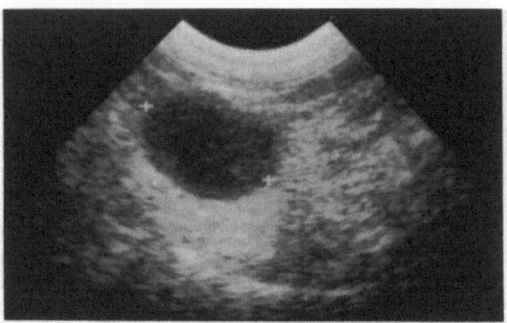

Fig. 4.1. Typical, well-marginated pleomorphic adenoma, less echogenic than the surrounding normal parotid tissue

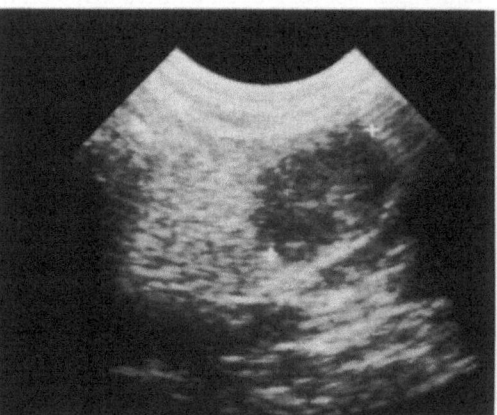

Fig. 4.2. Typical pleomorphic adenoma (18 mm between the two *crosses*)

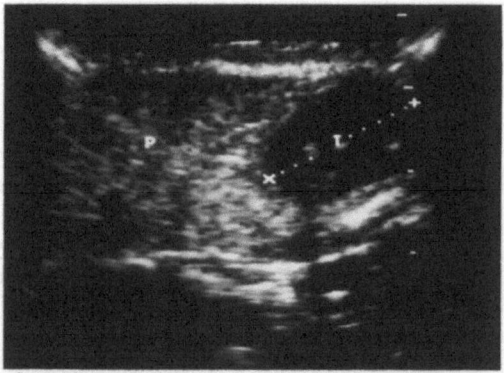

Fig. 4.3. Pleomorphic adenoma *(T)* (21 mm between the two *crosses*) distinctly demarcated from the normal parotid tissue

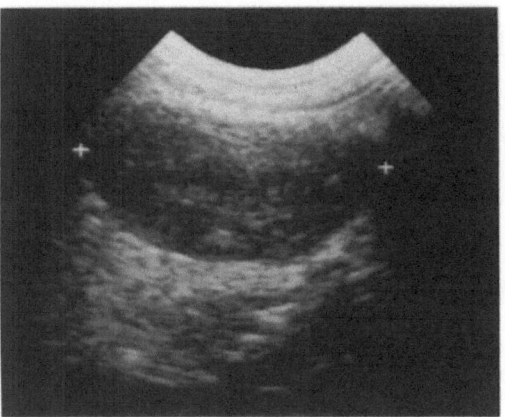

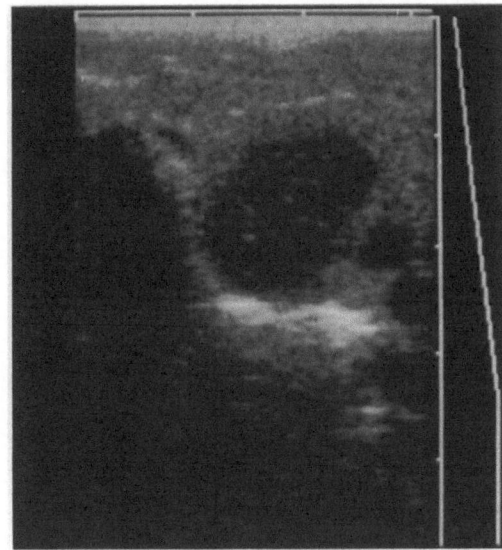

Fig. 4.4. Typical pleomorphic adenoma of the parotid gland (33 mm between the two *crosses*)

Fig. 4.6. Intraoperative sonogram showing the venous and arterial relations of a pleomorphic adenoma

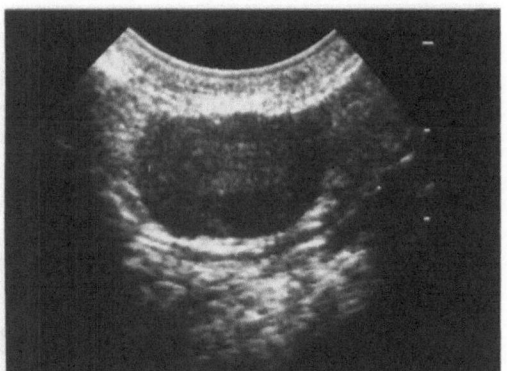

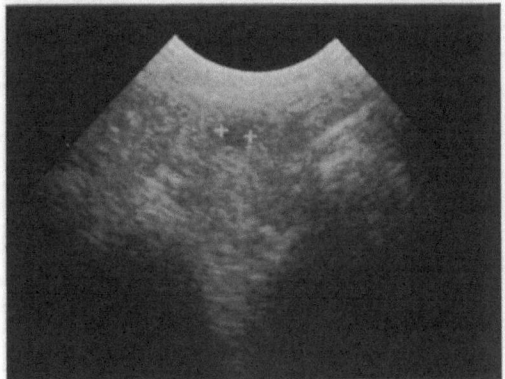

Fig. 4.5. Pleomorphic adenoma of the submandibular gland

Fig. 4.7. Small, nonpalpable pleomorphic adenoma not demonstrable by other imaging techniques (4 mm between the two *crosses*)

Certain tumors, and especially those larger than 3 cm, are prone to cystic and hemorrhagic degeneration which modifies their internal structure (Figs. 4.9 and 4.10). Degenerative changes are responsible for complex US images while extracapsular tumoral extension can be the source of ill-defined margins. Such sonographic features are suggestive of a neoplastic process, independent of the clinical history.

Total parotidectomy has only recently been adopted as the preferred surgical procedure for mixed tumors. Recurrent lesions continue to be seen in patients who were offered only partial surgical excision. US examination of patients operated on previously is hindered by the echogenic scar with an acoustic shadow and deep-seated tissue alterations which hamper interpretation (Fig. 4.11). Nevertheless, recurrent

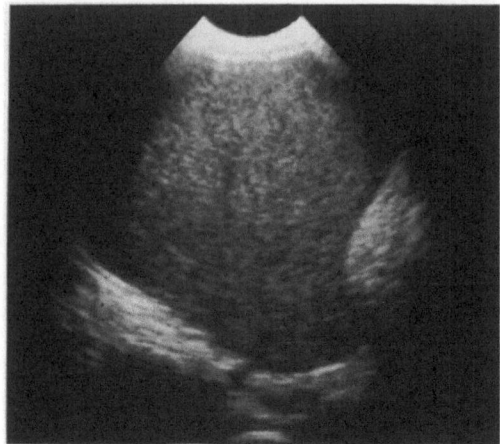

Fig. 4.8. Large (7 cm) pleomorphic adenoma of the parotid gland with a uniform echo pattern and well-defined margins

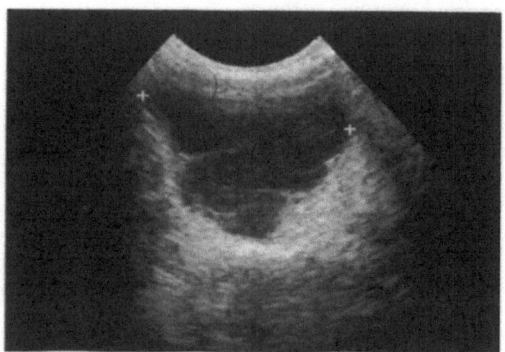

Fig. 4.9. Sharply defined pleomorphic adenoma with a discretely disorganized internal structure (29 mm between the two *crosses*)

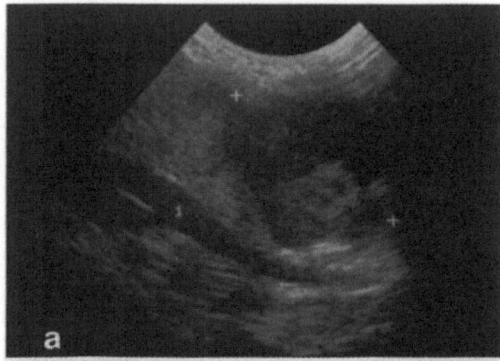

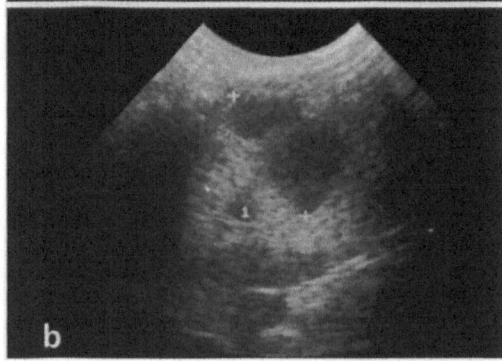

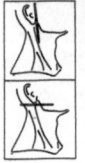
Fig. 4.10 a, b. Venous relations *(1)* of a pleomorphic adenoma; **a** sagittal scan, **b** transverse scan. The tumor is located some distance from the venous plane, and thus is not in contact with the facial nerve

lesions have the same ultrasonic pattern as "new" adenomas; only nearby, scar-related changes will appear suspicious owing to the complex US pattern they create.

As for all salivary gland swellings, the node-bearing areas of the neck must be examined sonographically with the patient supine. However, pleomorphic adenoma is not accompanied by cervical lymphadenopathy.

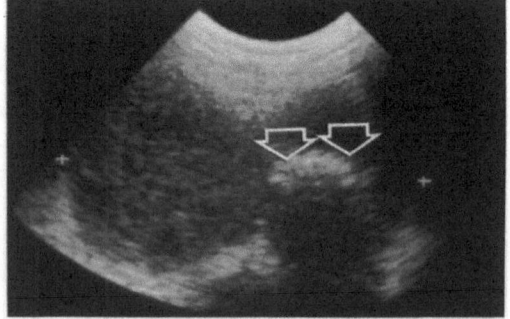

Fig. 4.11. Well-circumscribed recurrent pleomorphic adenoma 15 years after enucleation. The strongly echogenic area *(arrows)* corresponds to postoperative fibrosis (49 mm between the two *crosses*)

4.2.1.2 Cystadenoma Lymphomatosum (Adenolymphoma)

Also called Warthin's tumor, these lesions account for 6%–10% of all parotid tumors and affect males more often than females. The diagnosis is often suggested by the clinical picture, i.e., an elderly man with a swelling on the lower aspect of the parotid. Cystadenolymphoma of the submandibular gland is rare. This tumor has an excellent prognosis and almost never recurs; malignant degeneration is extremely rare. Only 5% of cases are bilateral.

Grossly, adenolymphoma corresponds to an encapsulated mass containing one or more cysts. Sonograms generally demonstrate a well-defined, anechogenic mass with posterior reinforcement, often at the lower pole of the parotid; distal echoes may be present. Such US features easily confirm the prospective clinical diagnosis (Figs. 4.12–4.14). In certain cases, multiple septa and the thickness of the intratumoral fluid set up discretely inhomogeneous echogenic images. This sonographic pattern is rare, and is usually interpreted as pleomorphic adenoma (Fig. 4.15). Scintigraphy is also required for such cases as detection of a warm zone will correct the diagnosis. Surgery may be indicated if the tumor is a source of discomfort; otherwise, continuing clinical and ultrasonographic surveillance will suffice.

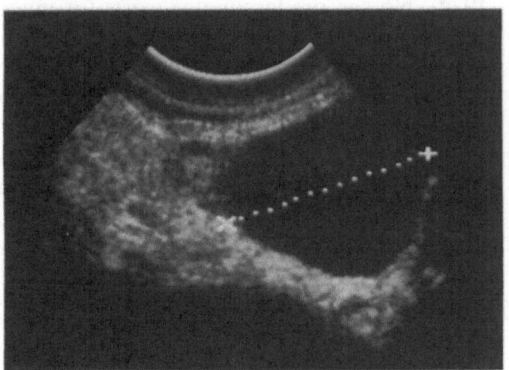

Fig. 4.12. Cystadenolymphoma of the lower pole of the parotid gland

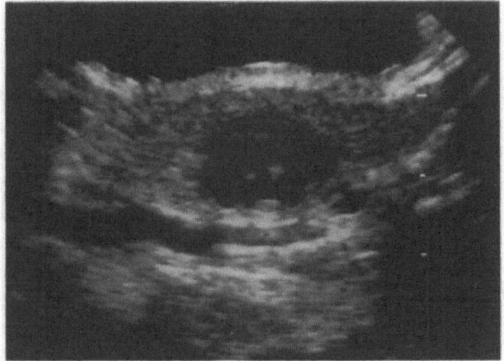

Fig. 4.14. Parotid cystadenolymphoma with internal echoes

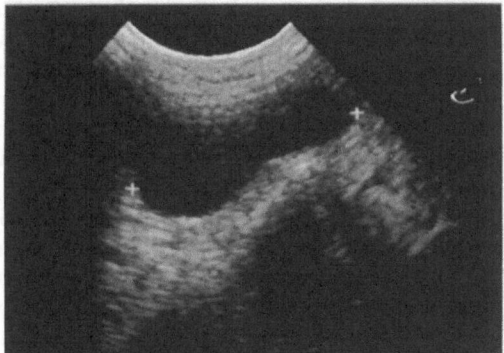

Fig. 4.13. Cystadenolymphoma of the anterior portion of the parotid

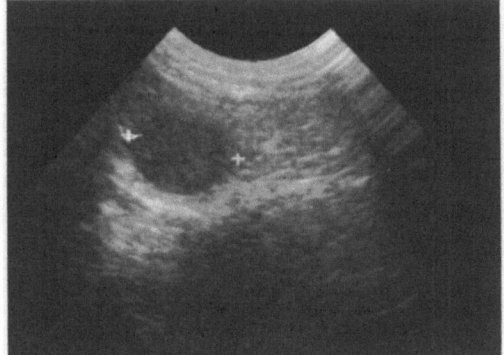

Fig. 4.15. Solid, echogenic parotid cystadenolymphoma

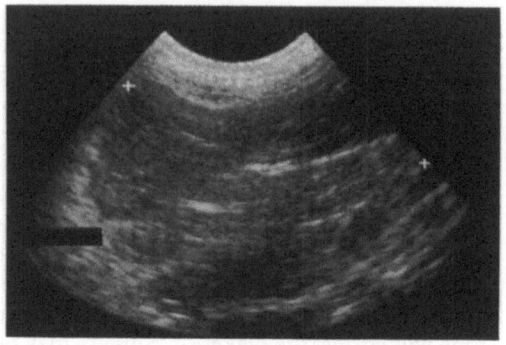

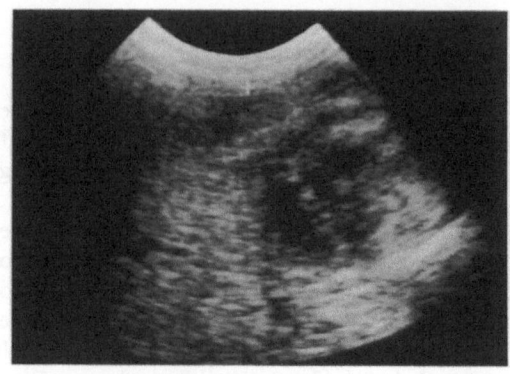

 Fig.4.16. Parotid lipoma

 Fig.4.17. Parotid carcinoma: US cannot evaluate deep spread

4.2.1.3 Benign Nonepithelial Salivary Gland Tumors

Tumors of this type arise within the glandular spaces from nonparenchymatous elements, and include lipomas, neurinomas, and vascular tumors. Lipoma presents as a discretely echogenic, sharply marginated soft mass. In one personal observation the particularly soft consistency of a superficial tumor suggested the diagnosis, which was confirmed by a CT scan demonstrating a mass of typical fat density (Fig. 4.16). Vascular tumors (hemangioma, lymphangioma) may have ill-defined margins, and they tend to have a complex US appearance. Most vascular tumors are seen in pediatric patients (Work 1977).

4.2.2 Malignant Salivary Gland Tumors

Just as they are the most common type of benign tumor, epithelial lesions are also the most frequent form of malignancy; metastases and lymphomas of the salivary glands are rare. Malignant epithelial tumors of the salivary glands represent 17% of all epithelial tumors.

4.2.2.1 Mucoepidermoid Carcinoma

Mucoepidermoid cancer accounts for 5%–10% of all salivary gland tumors, 80% of which affect the parotid gland (Thackray and Lucas

1974). No sex predominance exists for mucoepidermoid carcinoma, and it can occur at any age. Clinically, most mucoepidermoid carcinomas present as a slow-growing, firm or hard mass; only a small proportion grow rapidly and are obviously malignant clinically. The gross anatomy corresponds to a nonencapsulated or only partly encapsulated tumor with a marked tendency to infiltrate adjacent tissues.

Small diameter tumors corresponding to early lesions can be differentiated sonographically from masses with a diameter greater than 2 cm. However, US cannot determine the benign or malignant nature of small (<2 cm), seemingly encapsulated masses because the resolution is not high enough to detect modifications in the echo pattern or lesion margins. Larger tumors may have a more complex internal pattern, but the best indication of their infiltrative nature is the absence of sharply defined margins. Except for cases treated previously by surgery, any breach in tumoral margins must be considered suspicious of malignancy. Advanced lesions are sonographically complex, occasionally with anechogenic zones secondary to necrosis or hemorrhage; the exact margins of the tumor cannot be determined. CT examination is indispensable for such cases. The diagnosis of mucoepidermoid carcinoma is usually made clinically, and US is basically indicated for the detection of cervical node metastases (Fig. 4.17).

4.2.2.2 Acinic Cell Tumors

Acinic cell tumors account for less than 3% of all parotid tumors. They may be confused clinically with a pleomorphic adenoma or present the typical features of malignancy. The malignant potential of these tumors is comparable to that of mucoepidermoid tumors. The gross anatomy corresponds to a solid tumor that may contain scattered cystic zones. Apart from cases characterized by infiltration, acinic cell tumors generally take the form of a well-circumscribed homogeneous nodule which suggests a diagnosis of pleomorphic adenoma.

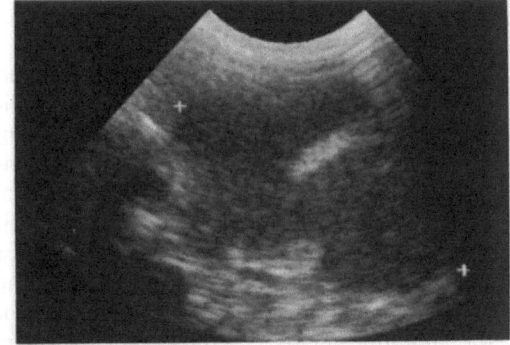

 Fig. 4.18. Parotid cylindroma

4.2.2.3 Carcinoma

Carcinomas represent the majority of malignant salivary gland tumors; cylindromas are the most prevalent type (Spiro et al. 1982).

Cylindromas, or adenoid cystic carcinomas, account for approximately 3% of all parotid tumors and 15%–17% of all submandibular gland tumors (Eneroth 1971; Thackray and Lucas 1974). These solitary, freely movable, rounded tumors may be accompanied by pain or facial paralysis. They most commonly affect women over 40 years of age. Although these well-defined masses appear homogeneous on gross inspection, histologic examination reveals infiltration of the surrounding tissues, and in particular the perineural structures. This last point is particularly important as facial paralysis is a constant feature of cylindromas.

Like other cancers, cylindromas sonographically resemble benign tumors when small. Even large lesions have no US features that are indicative of cylindroma rather than another form of cancer (Figs. 4.18 and 4.19). This insufficiency of imaging studies is particularly regrettable because, in addition to the actual prognosis, paralysis is almost constant following surgery. Indeed, even small cylindromas that appear well circumscribed at gross examination rapidly infiltrate both proximal nerve fibers and the distant branches of the facial nerve. Only extemporaneous histologic examination can accurately determine the extent of local or distant invasion, which occurs frequently and requires sacrifice of the facial nerve.

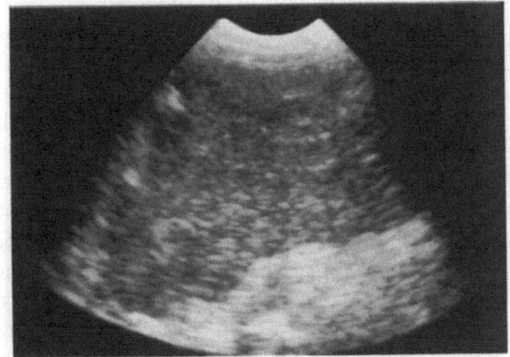

 Fig. 4.19. Parotid cylindroma

The other carcinomas encountered in the salivary glands are either more or less undifferentiated cancers or epidermoid carcinomas. Once these tumors attain 2 cm, sonographic anomalies in the tumor's margins suffice to suggest malignancy. US is of limited interest for large lesions as the diagnosis will have already been made clinically, and evaluation of spread to deep structures is usually difficult. CT is indicated for analysis of in-depth tumor spread, and ultrasonography for exploration of the cervical lymph node-bearing areas.

4.2.2.4 Nonepithelial Salivary Gland Tumors

Nonepithelial tumors are rare, and correspond to metastases and lymphomas. Aside from direct tumoral spread from an adjacent lesion, the most common causes of metastasis are malignant melanoma and epidermoid carcinoma. Lesions secondary to hematogenous dissemination, such as occurs in melanoma, manifest as well-circumscribed nodules, and only the clinical context and the rapid development of the nodule suggest a metastatic etiology (Fig. 4.20).

Epidermoid carcinoma may result from lymphatic disease dissemination, for example, from a pharyngeal cancer. Along with the obvious clinical context, the presence of cervical nodal masses is helpful for diagnosis.

Lymphomas are essentially represented by non-Hodgkin's lymphomas (Figs. 4.21 and 4.22). Salivary sites of lymphoma are extremely rare, however, and only some 100 cases of nonnodal primary salivary lymphoma have been reported in the literature (Bruneton et al. 1982). Apart from lymphomatous intraparotid nodes, both primary and secondary lymphoma of the parotid gland are exceedingly rare; the sonographic image is strongly hypoechogenic or even anechogenic, with posterior reinforcement. If ultrasonography fails to detect any cervical node involvement, the usual diagnosis is pleomorphic adenoma or cystadenolymphoma (for lesions at the lower pole of the parotid gland).

4.2.3 Related Tumors

These very rare tumors are described only briefly; certain are described in more detail in other chapters.

Cystic lesions of the salivary glands are uncommon. The majority occur in the parotid gland, but even then they account for only 2%–5% of all parotid lesions (Rice 1984). Salivary cysts may be either congenital or acquired. Congenital cysts derive from the first branchial groove and are generally diagnosed in infancy; they are visualized by US as well-limited, anechogenic forms. The possible origins of acquired cysts include a neoplastic process, benign lymphoepithelial lesion, trauma, parotitis, and cal-

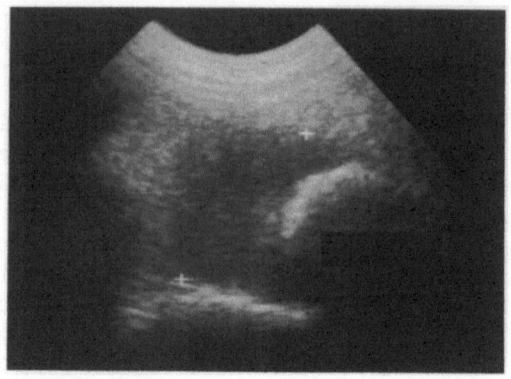

Fig. 4.20. Parotid metastasis from thyroid cancer (23 mm between the two *crosses*)

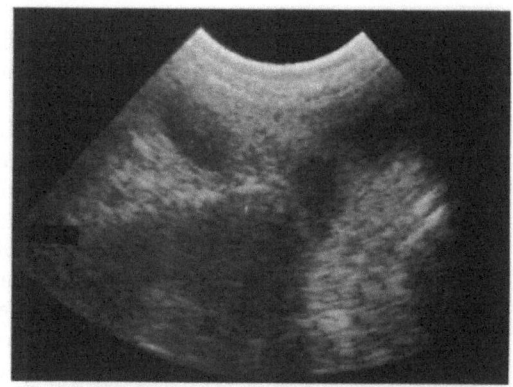

Fig. 4.21. Large lymphomatous parotid tumor

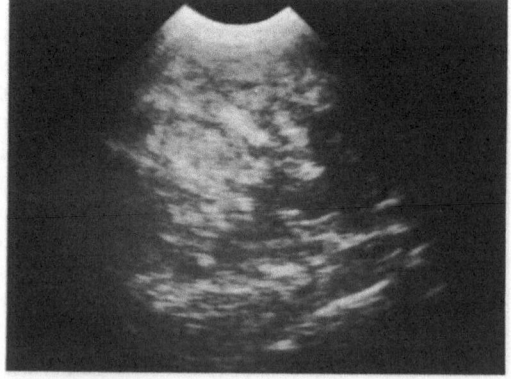

Fig. 4.22. Infiltrative primary lymphoma of the parotid

culi. Mucus-retention cysts, true cysts with an epithelial lining, form in reaction to partial duct obstruction (complete duct obstruction causes glandular atrophy). Mucoceles are not true cysts and tend to involve the minor salivary glands; sites of predilection include the lips, buccal mucosa, and the ventral tongue (Work 1977).

Pseudotumors actually correspond to nodular involution of one of several lesion types, including chronic lithiasic parotitis, tuberculosis, and benign lymphoepithelial lesions.

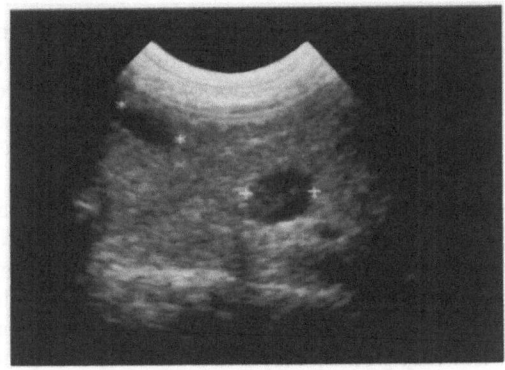

Fig. 4.23. Strongly hypoechogenic, lymphomatous intraparotid nodes

4.2.4 Multinodular Lesions

If nodular masses are defined as lesions with a minimum diameter of 5 mm (which eliminates chronic inflammatory pathologies), multinodular lesions almost always correspond to malignant nodes. As indicated in Chap. 1, extracapsular and intraglandular nodes are associated with both the parotid and the submandibular glands. When enlarged, these nodes appear oval or rounded, and their uniform echo pattern is less echogenic than the normal gland. A solitary intraglandular nodal mass may be confused with a benign tumor (Bruneton et al. 1985). Multiple lesions are the rule, however, and transverse diameters usually range from 5 to 20 mm. Multinodular lesions have several possible etiologies:

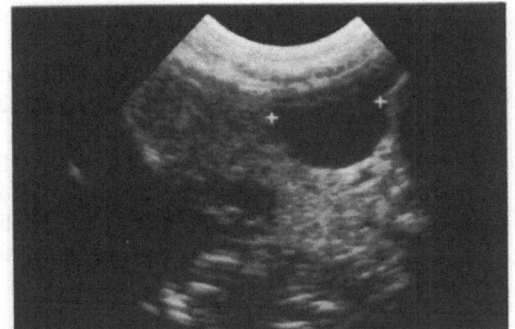

Fig. 4.24. Strongly hypoechogenic, lymphomatous submaxillary nodes

- *Malignant lymphoma*. Primary lymphoma of the parotid is unusual, but intraparotid lymphomatous nodes are fairly often associated with lymphomatous cervical nodes. By contrast, solitary intraparotid nodal masses are generally not lymphomatous if there is no concomitant cervical lymphadenopathy. Multiple salivary gland involvement by lymphomatous nodes is not uncommon and is always associated with cervical node involvement (Figs. 4.23–4.25).
- *Cancer of the tongue* has usually already been diagnosed by physical examination when ultrasonography is employed to detect swelling of one or both submaxillary regions. On rare occasions, discovery of enlarged submaxillary nodes leads to diagnosis of a hitherto unsuspected tumor of the floor of the mouth or the tongue. Discovery of uni-

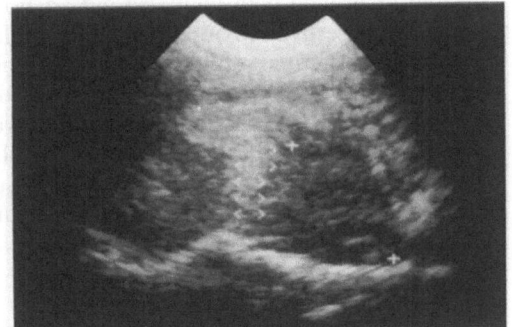

Fig. 4.25. Echogenic, lymphomatous intraparotid nodes

or bilateral multinodular submaxillary images should prompt a search for cancer of the tongue or the floor of the mouth as well as exploration of the subjacent lateral neck to detect possible cervical nodal involvement.

- *Sarcoiditis* rarely manifests clinically as a salivary gland tumor; when it does, the favored site is the submandibular gland. By revealing multinodular disease, ultrasonography rules out a diagnosis of a primary tumor of the salivary glands, and, if there is no known context of sarcoidosis, surgical exploration is recommended.

- *Oncocytosis* is a very rare pathology which, contrary to the preceding three etiologies, does not affect the lymph nodes. It may be localized to a single salivary gland or involve several glands simultaneously. Oncocytosis should be suspected when multinodular lesions are imaged in several salivary glands and no enlarged jugulocarotid nodes are found. Aspiration biopsy is usually sufficient for diagnosis as these lesions have no malignant potential. US is indicated for follow-up purposes and, to be complete, must visualize all of the salivary glands (Figs. 4.26 and 4.27).

Aside from those acute or chronic infectious processes already detected clinically, US of the neck can determine the etiology of multinodular salivary gland lesions at least 5 mm in diameter as a function of lesion location prior to surgical findings. Multinodular disease of a single gland associated with jugulocarotid adenopathies is suggestive of lymphoma; submaxillary involvement requires clinical and sonographic explorations of the oral cavity in a search for a tumor. Multinodular lesions in several salivary glands accompanied by cervical node involvement almost always indicate lymphoma. Solitary multinodular lesions without associated cervical adenopathies suggest oncocytosis.

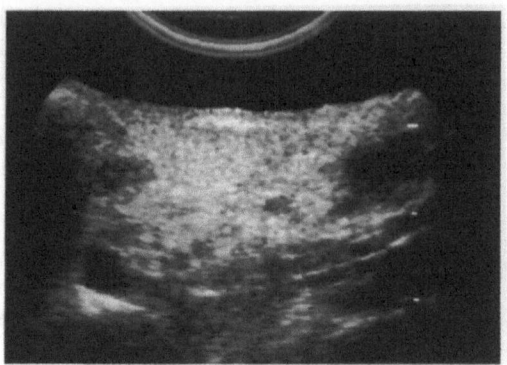

Fig. 4.26. Parotid oncocytosis (nodules range in size from 3 to 20 mm)

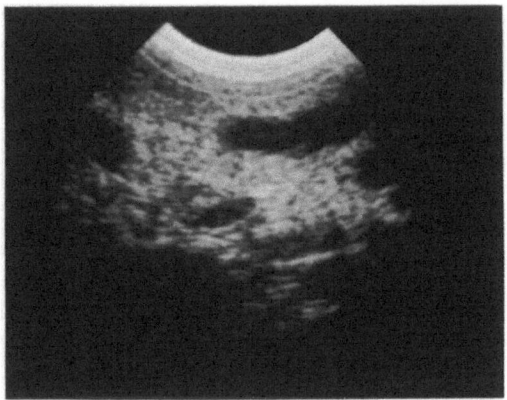

Fig. 4.27. Parotid oncocytosis (nodules range in size from 5 to 20 mm)

4.2.5 Value and Limitations of Ultrasonography for Salivary Gland Tumors

4.2.5.1 Topographic and Etiologic Limitations

US exploration of salivary gland neoplasms is hampered by several problems related to the topography and etiology of the lesions. It cannot visualize the entire parotid gland; the portion posterior to the ascending ramus of the mandible and the pharyngeal parotid extension in particular are inaccessible to US. Tumoral relations with the nerve plexus of the parotid cannot be evaluated by US because the facial nerve is not visible; however, a superficial no-

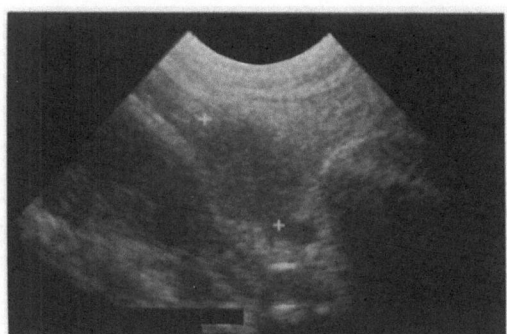

Fig.4.28. Parotid cancer with a benign US appearance revealed by cervical nodal masses and hepatic metastases

4.2.5.2 Value of Ultrasonography

US is a simple, rapid, and noninvasive examination that lasts only a few minutes, yet can correctly differentiate benign tumors from malignant processes in nearly 80% of cases. Diagnosis relies not only on the echo pattern and margins (well-or ill-defined) of salivary gland lesions, but also on systematic exploration of the cervical lymph node-bearing areas, preferably with a high frequency transducer. Aside from high quality preliminary results obtained with MRI using surface coils, no other currently available imaging technique, particularly neither sialography nor CT, appears superior to US for etiological diagnosis.

dule less than 3 cm in greatest dimension will be located at some distance from this nerve. Actually, the insufficiency of imaging studies, and particularly US, to analyze connections with the facial nerve affects only those rare larger lesions, which tend to be malignant. However, certain clinical features (facial paralysis) associated with large or malignant tumors do allow assessment of their involvement with the facial nerve. The last topographic drawback of US concerns the impossibility of evaluating the spread of large tumors to deep structures.

As mentioned, false negative errors of malignancy can be caused by small encapsulated tumors such as mucoepidermoid cancers or cylindromas (Fig.4.28). Although they are rare, solitary intraglandular nodal masses and metastases also generally appear sonographically benign. False positive errors occur with very advanced or recurrent mixed tumors. Previous surgery may have altered the internal structure of the lesion, creating false images of parietal irregularities.

Except for evaluation of the spread of large and probably malignant tumors to deep structures, which can be studied advantageously by CT, none of the shortcomings of US seem to be compensated by other available imaging techniques.

4.2.6 Protocol for the Exploration of Salivary Gland Masses

Not all salivary gland swellings are tumors, and when doubt persists after physical examination US can easily affirm or confirm the diagnosis of tumor (Bruneton et al. 1983). Except for gland swelling caused by the presence of multiple nodular lesions, salivary tumors tend to be solitary. Small lesions (less than 3 cm in diameter) with well-defined margins demonstrated sonographically within healthy surrounding tissue probably do not require further examination by other imaging techniques prior to surgery, whether or not US detects cervical node enlargement.

When sonography fails to define the margins of a lesion, and especially if normal peripheral tissue cannot be imaged, this data must be obtained by CT. If high resolution CT equipment is available, sialography is probably unnecessary, although it can be performed if doubt still persists as to the limits or origin of the tumor. By contrast, if an older and thus slower and less effective CT scanner is used, sialography can be an interesting complementary means of obtaining answers to questions left unsolved by US.

US examination of the submaxillary region in patients who have undergone surgery involves no great difficulties; images that are discretely echogenic relative to the adjacent muscles will correspond to local fibrosis. By contrast, sonographic exploration of the posttreatment parotid is not always satisfactory (Fig. 4.29). If doubt persists after physical examination, and in particular after exeresis of a malignant tumor, CT is required because recurrence may be deep-seated, in a parapharyngeal or even endocranial site (Figs. 4.30–4.32).

Overall, ultrasonography has replaced sialography as the procedure of choice for initial investigation of a salivary gland tumor. In nearly three-quarters of all cases, its findings are sufficient to serve as the basis for a therapeutic decision.

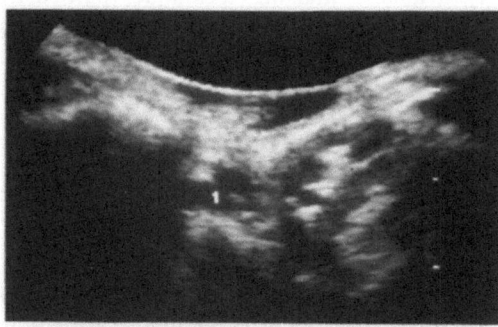

 Fig. 4.29. Normal appearance after parotidectomy: the scar tissue is echogenic and the external carotid artery *(1)* occupies a more superficial position

Fig. 4.31. Recurrence of a mixed tumor in the retromandibular region (not visible with US) detected after discovery of an endobuccal mass

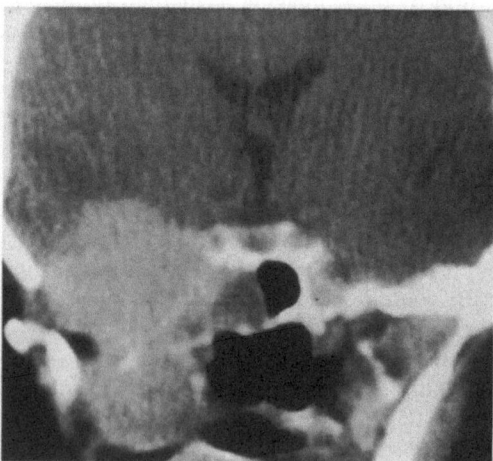

Fig. 4.30. Recurrence of a parotid cancer in the homolateral temporal fossa

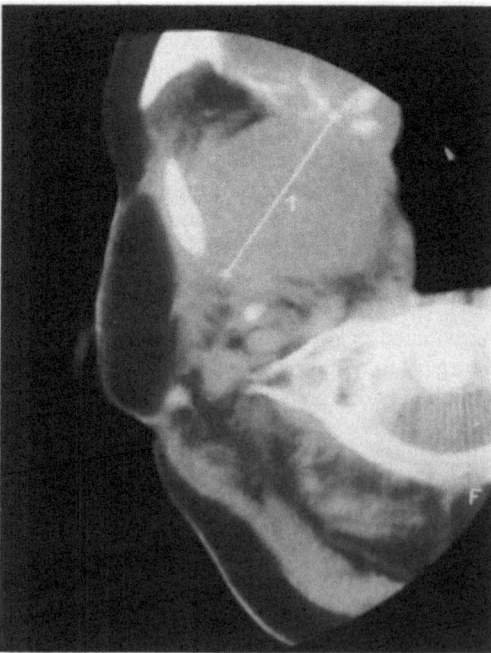

Fig. 4.32. Recurrence of a parotid cancer in the retromandibular region (not visible with US)

4.3 Inflammatory Disease

Only four types of inflammatory disorders will be described: acute suppurative sialadenitis, chronic recurrent sialadenitis, Sjögren's syndrome, and viroses (Mason and Chisholm 1975; Work and Hecht 1968).

4.3.1 Acute Suppurative Sialadenitis

The incidence of this pathology has decreased considerably over the past few years; its etiology is basically postoperative, especially after GI tract procedures. An ascending bacterial infection is the predominant cause; hyposialosis, xerostomia, and immunodepression are all associated factors.

Regardless of whether the disease develops gradually or occurs suddenly, there is usually an initial inflammatory phase characterized by edema and pain during which the orifice of the parotid duct is red and contains pus. Diagnosis is made clinically, and imaging procedures pro-vide no determinant information; ultrasonography is difficult to perform because of the pain involved, and can only demonstrate diffuse enlargement. Administration of antibiotics generally prevents evolution toward the second phase, suppuration; if it does occur, US can demonstrate a well-limited, more or less anechogenic mass associated with painful enlargement of the cervical nodes (Fig. 4.33).

4.3.2 Chronic Recurrent Sialadenitis

Chronic recurrent sialadenitis is associated with decreased secretion of saliva and subsequent stasis, affecting children as well as adults. A history of regional infectious and lithiasic episodes is common. US provides no useful information, and sialography is required for this pathology.

Opacification of early forms in children demonstrates small intraductal cystic ectasia; US and other imaging procedures are not indicated, except perhaps for investigation of acute episodes when abscess formation is feared. For advanced forms, however, US can demonstrate diffuse ductal dilatation (Fig. 4.34).

4.3.3 Sjögren's Syndrome (Sicca Syndrome)

Sjögren's syndrome is a common autoimmune disease seen almost exclusively in women; average age by onset is 50 years or more. Patients

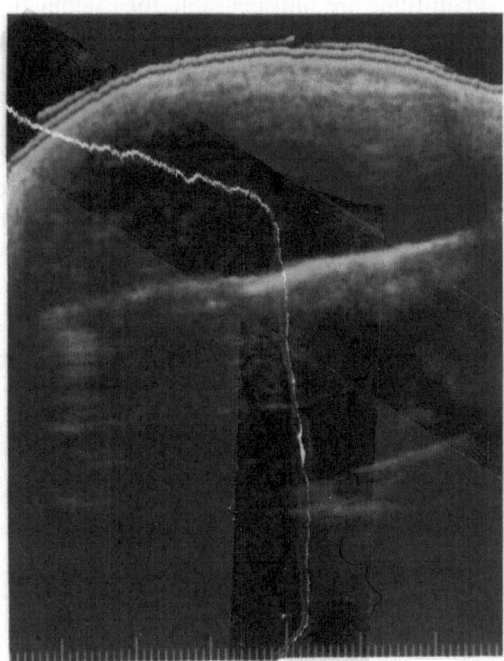

Fig. 4.33. Parotid abscess

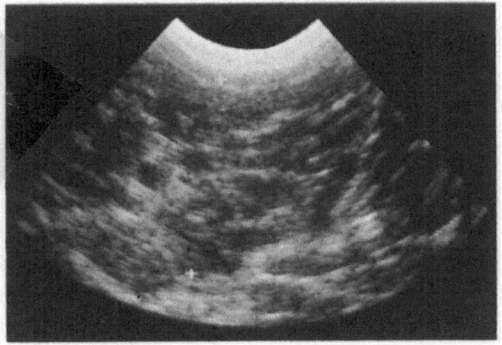

Fig. 4.34. Diffuse, bilateral intraductal cystic ectasia of the parotid gland in a 3-year-old child

may present with xerostomia or hyposialosis, xerophthalmia, dryness of the nasal mucosae, and occasionally parotid swelling. Sialography is particularly indicated because of the parallelism between the syndrome's radiologic appearance and histological severity (Shearn 1977). In its early stages, it may manifest solely as punctate opacification of the parenchyma. As the disease progresses, extravasation may be observed through the disorganized ductal epithelium; such images are highly suggestive of the diagnosis. US can detect swelling when it exists, but neither it nor CT can visualize the ducts except in very advanced cases. Scintigraphy is an excellent procedure for global evaluation of all of the salivary glands and especially for monitoring response to therapy. Like all benign lymphoepithelial lesions, Sjögren's syndrome may be associated with lymphoma (Rice 1984), and US surveillance of the cervical nodes is thus recommended.

4.3.4 Viral Infections

Mumps (infectious parotitis) is the most frequent cause of parotid gland swelling. Diagnosis is made clinically and no imaging studies are required; US can only demonstrate painful unilateral or bilateral parotid enlargement accompanied by nodal enlargement.

On the whole, inflammatory disease of the salivary glands is generally diagnosed clinically and biologically. Sialography is the most useful examination technique; ultrasonography is indicated only to verify the presence or absence of an abscess or tumoral mass.

4.4 Nonneoplastic, Noninflammatory Salivary Gland Pathologies

4.4.1 Trauma

Injury to the parotid gland accounts for most cases of salivary tissue trauma, and is the only circumstance involving therapeutic problems because of the other important anatomic structures in the area (external carotid artery, facial nerve, parotid duct). Assessment of parotid injuries is probably best performed with CT. If doubt persists as to the possibility of parotid

duct damage, sialograms provide the best anatomic detail. US is of limited interest for traumatic pathologies, particularly if a fistula is present. On rare occasions a sialocele or a hematoma can be validly explored by US.

4.4.2 Sialolithiasis

Sialolithiasis is much more common in the submandibular gland than in the parotid; parotid stones are usually not detected until complications, especially infection, occur (Epker 1972; Suleiman and Hobsley 1980). Single stones account for three-fourths of all cases affecting the major salivary glands; multiple calculi affecting several glands occur in only 3% of cases (Rice 1984). Nearly all submandibular stones are radiopaque whereas most parotid calculi are radiolucent. Sialoliths can be the origin of an ascending ductal infection which may spread to the glandular tissue. Clinical features include recurrent swelling of the affected gland and pain, which is often exacerbated by eating. Submandibular stones are frequently palpable.

Plain films are indispensable for examination of uncomplicated cases. For the parotid gland, plain anteroposterior radiographs coupled with an intrabuccal film succeed in demonstrating a calculus in 75% of cases. If radiography is negative, sialography almost always reveals the cause of lithiasis (Rice 1984). According to Hajek et al. (1984) ultrasonography successfully detects calculi in 91% of cases.

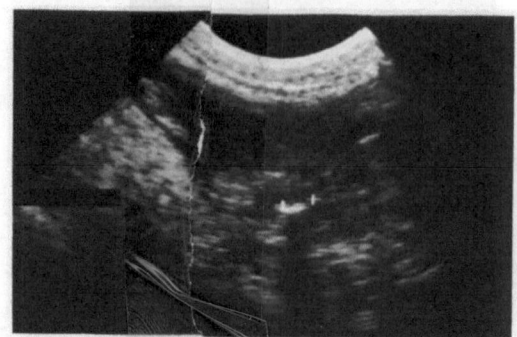

Fig. 4.35. Submandibular calculus (4 mm between the two *crosses*) presenting as a strongly echogenic image with a posterior acoustic shadow

When ductal cannulation is impossible, ultrasound may be able to detect a radiotransparent calculus, and can roughly evaluate the condition of the suprajacent parenchyma (Fig. 4.35). For stones located within the gland tissue, accurate anatomic localization by US allows lithotripsy to be offered as a therapeutic alternative. Sialolithiasis can be complicated by infection and ductal lesions (ulceration, stricture) (Rice 1984).

4.4.3 Sialadenosis

Sialadenosis is a general term that refers to any nonneoplastic and noninflammatory enlargement of a salivary gland. Swelling is usually asymptomatic and the diagnosis is clinical. When the diagnosis remains doubtful, and also for severe swelling, US can affirm enlargement and the absence of tumor. Nutrition-related factors are the most common systemic etiologies: excessive starch intake in the diet, alcoholism, severe malnutrition, diabetes, gout (Fig. 4.36). Drug-induced (toxic) and allergic sialomegaly are much rarer.

Sialadenosis generally has a favorable prognosis, and the involved gland returns to normal as soon as the systemic cause is corrected.

4.5 Conclusion

To conclude, the most valuable use of ultrasonography for salivary gland pathologies concerns the investigation of tumors; in these cases, ultrasound exploration of the involved gland must always be extended to include examination of the lateral side of the neck to detect any lymph node involvement. It is helpful when doubt persists as to the existence of a tumor or an abscess in connection with an acute inflammatory pathology. Although inflammatory disease is best investigated by sialography, sialolithiasis can be advantageously studied by US.

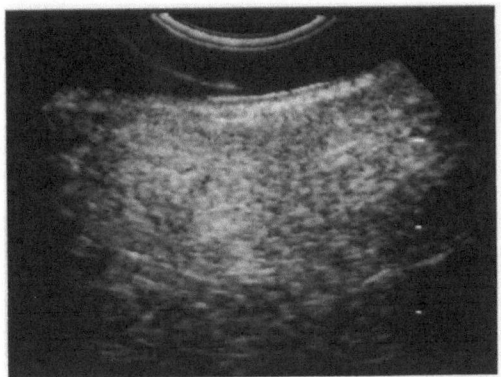

Fig. 4.36. Sialadenosis of alcoholic origin causing diffuse parotid enlargement

4.6 References

Baker S, Ossoinig KG (1977) Ultrasonic evaluation of salivary glands. Trans Am Acad Ophthalmol Otolaryngol 84: 750–762

Ballerini G, Mantero M, Sbrocca M (1984) Ultrasonic patterns of parotid masses. JCU 12: 273–277

Bellina PV Jr (1982) Diagnostic use of ultrasound in sialolithiasis of the parotid gland. J La State Med Soc 134: 79–82

Bruneton JN, Roux P (1984) Tumeurs des glandes salivaires. In: Bruneton JN, Matter D, Benozio M, Senecail B (eds) Echographie en pathologie tumorale de l'adulte. Masson, Paris, pp 11–15

Bruneton JN, Fenart D, Vallicioni J, Demard F (1980) Séméiologie échographique des tumeurs de la parotide. A propos de 40 observations. J Radiol 61: 151–154

Bruneton JN, Caramella E, Boublil JL, Roux P, Abbes M, Demard F (1982) Echographic aspects of thyroid and parotid localizations in non-Hodgkin's lymphomas. Rofo 136: 530–533

Bruneton JN, Sicart M, Roux P, Pastaud P, Nicolau A, Delorme G (1983) Indications for ultrasonography in parotid pathologies. Rofo 138: 22–24

Bruneton JN, Caramella E, Roux P, Fenart J, Manzino JJ (1985) Comparison of ultrasonographic and histological findings for multinodular lesions of the salivary glands. Europ J Radiol 5: 295–296

Bryan RN, Miller RH, Ferreyro RI, Sessions RB (1982) Computed tomography of the major salivary glands. AJR 139: 547–554

Calcaterra TC, Hemengay WG, Hansen GC, Hanafee WN (1977) The value of sialography in the diagnosis of parotid tumours. A clinicopathological correlation. Arch Otol 103: 727–729

Conn IG, Wiesenfeld D, Ferguson MM (1983) The anatomy of the facial nerve in relation to CT/sialography of the parotid gland. Br J Radiol 56: 901–905

Einstein RAJ (1966) Sialography in the differential diagnosis of parotid masses. Surg Gynecol Obstet 122: 1079–1083

Eneroth CM (1971) Salivary gland tumors in the parotid gland, submandibular gland, and the palate region. Cancer 27: 1415–1418

Epker BN (1972) Obstructive and inflammatory diseases of the major salivary glands. Oral Surg 33: 2–27

Eyjolfsson O, Nordshus T, Dahl T (1984) Sialography and CT-sialography in the diagnosis of parotid masses. Acta Radiol (Diagn) (Stockh) 25: 361–364

Gates GA (1971) Radiosialographic aspects of salivary gland disorders. Laryngoscope 82: 115–130

Hajek PC, Wittich GR, Tuerk R, Kumpan W, Canigiani G (1984) High-resolution sonography and sialography in sialadenitis and sialolithiasis. Radiology 153 (P): 82

Kushner DC, Weber AL (1978) Sialography of salivary gland tumours with fibroscopy and tomography. AJR 130: 941–944

McGahan JP, Walter JP, Bernstein L (1984) Evaluation of the parotid gland. Comparison of sialography, non-contrast computed tomography, and CT sialography. Radiology 152: 453–458

Mancuso AA, Hanafee WN (1982) Computed tomography of the head and neck. Williams and Wilkins, Baltimore

Mason DK, Chisholm DM (1975) Salivary glands in health and disease. Saunders, Philadelphia

Neiman H, Phillips JF, Jaques DA, Brown TL (1976) Ultrasound of the parotid gland. JCU 4: 11–13

Ohrt JH, Shafer RB (1982) An atlas of salivary gland disorders. Clin Nucl Med 7: 370–376

Pickrell KL, Trought WS, Shearin JC (1978) The use of ultrasound to localize calculi within the parotid gland. Ann Plast Surg 1: 542–546

Rice DH (1984) Advances in diagnosis and management of salivary gland diseases. West J Med 140: 238–249

Schmitt G, Lehmann G, Stroetges MW, Wehmer W, Reinecke V, Teske HJ, Rottinger EM (1976) The diagnostic value of sialography and scintigraphy in salivary gland disease. Br J Radiol 49: 326–329

Shearn MA (1977) Sjogren's syndrome. Med Clin North Am 61: 271–272

Som PM, Biller HF (1980) The combined CT sialogram. Radiology 135: 387–390

Spiro RH, Huvos AG, Strong EW (1982) Adenocarcinoma of salivary origin. Clinicopathologic study of 204 patients. Am J Surg 144: 423–431

Suleiman SI, Hobsley M (1980) Radiological appearances of parotid duct calculi. Br J Surg 67: 879–880

Thackray AC, Lucas RB (1974) Tumors of the major salivary glands. Atlas of tumor pathology, 2nd series, Fasc 10. AFIP, Washington DC

Work WP (1977) Cysts and congenital lesions of the parotid gland. Otolaryngol Clin North Am 10: 339–343

Work WP, Hecht DW (1968) Non-neoplastic lesions of the parotid gland. Ann Otol Rhinol Laryngol 77: 462–467

5 Cervical Lymph Nodes

J.-N. BRUNETON AND F. NORMAND

Owing to the lymphatic richness of the cervical region (cf. Chap. 1), one or more enlarged lymph nodes are commonly present in both inflammatory and tumoral pathologies. The indications and shortcomings of ultrasound (US) for thyroid, parathyroid, and salivary gland investigations have been recognized for some time. By contrast, the value of sonographic studies for exploration of the cervical lymph nodes has only been established recently, as a consequence of the more widespread availability of high resolution, real-time US equipment. A decade ago, analyses of the comparative value of clinical and surgical findings commonly pointed out the insufficiency of physical examination, and emphasized the need for surgical dissection, especially for ENT cancer patients (Jesse and Fletcher 1963; MacGavran et al. 1961; Manfredi and Jacobelli 1975; Martis et al. 1979; Mustard and Rosen 1963; Sako et al. 1964). Currently, the emphasis in reports has shifted to the utility of ultrasound for both disease staging and follow-up of patients with head and neck cancer or lymphoma.

5.1 Ultrasonography of the Cervical Lymph Nodes

Despite their solid US pattern, normal lymph nodes cannot be visualized sonographically. Even large lipomatous nodes are not visible with US because their fat component is indistinguishable from the subcutaneous tissue. Only enlarged nodes are sonographically visible because these round or oval masses are globally hypoechogenic relative to the surrounding tissue.

5.1.1 US Pattern

5.1.1.1 Lymphoma and Metastatic Disease

The sonographic image theoretically reflects the internal architecture of the node. The non-Hodgkin's lymphoma node consists of homogeneous cellular sheets, and the US beam thus encounters few interfaces; this explains why these nodes are frequently hypoechogenic and

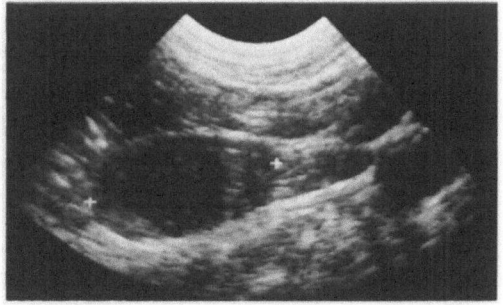

Fig. 5.1. Non-Hodgkin's lymphoma spinal chain node

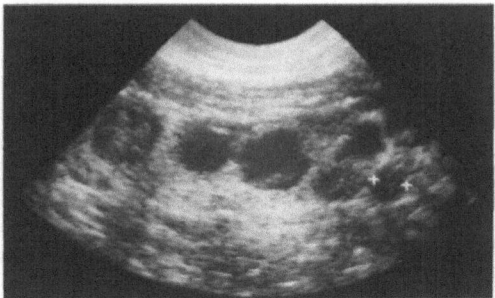

Fig. 5.2. Small jugulocarotid non-Hodgkin's lymphoma nodes (5 mm between the two *crosses*)

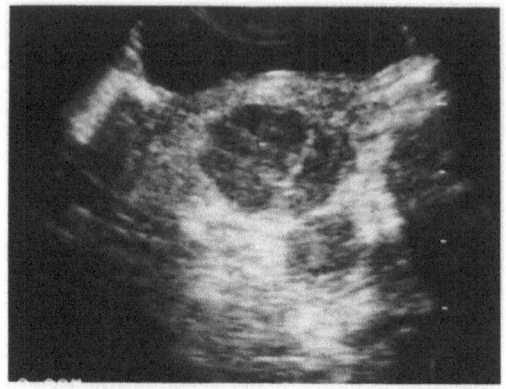

Fig. 5.3. Solid metastatic nodes

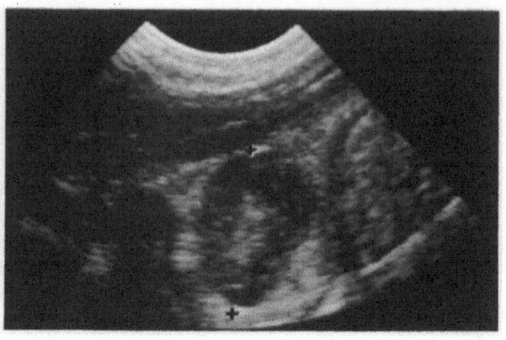

Fig. 5.5. Metastatic cervical nodes (21 mm between the two *crosses*)

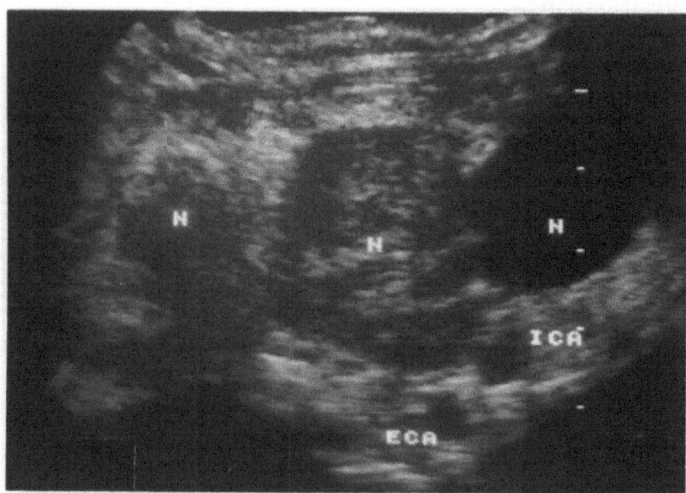

Fig. 5.4. Metastatic nodes *(N)* anterior to the internal carotid *(ICA)* and external carotid arteries *(ECA)*

may even exhibit posterior reinforcement (Figs. 5.1 and 5.2). In certain instances, the gain must be increased to demonstrate the lesion's solid nature. By contrast, both metastatic nodes and Hodgkin's disease nodes may be composed of tumoral areas adjacent to normal nodal zones, and the numerous interfaces which result explain why the US image is more echogenic (Figs. 5.3–5.5).

5.1.1.2 Nonspecificity of the US Pattern

Although non-Hodgkin's lymphoma nodes tend to be strongly hypoechogenic, not all metastatic nodes are solid or have a complex US appearance. US characterization of nodal architecture thus connot be used as the basis for either diagnosis. Even detection of a signal in Doppler ultrasound studies is not specific for either diagnosis (Mountford and Atkinson 1979).

5.1.1.3 Inflammatory Nodes

When located in a position allowing thorough analysis, enlarged inflammatory nodes may also appear hypoechogenic. There are no specific US patterns which permit differentiation of inflammatory etiologies from tumoral processes (Figs. 5.6–5.8).

5.1.1.4 Influence of Cervical Irradiation on Nodal Architecture

In addition to inducing regression in lesion size, cervical irradiation can also alter the internal architecture of the lymph nodes. The resultant discretely inhomogeneous, hyperechogenic structure may even progress to calcification, in which case the US image is strongly echogenic, with a posterior acoustic shadow (Figs. 5.9 and 5.10).

5.1.2 Measurement of Node Size

Accurate evaluation of enlarged lymph nodes requires measurement of their transverse diameter. The longitudinal diameter is less helpful as normal nodes exhibit considerable variation in this dimension. Node measurements for staging and follow-up purposes must therefore be made from transverse scans.

5.1.2.1 ENT Cancer

Based on the findings of various anatomic studies, nodes with a transverse diameter over 8 mm can generally be considered metastatic; smaller nodes are apt to have an inflammatory etiology. Of course, this 8-mm cutoff point is merely an artificial statistical creation whose use will result in both false negative and false positive errors of metastasis, but it remains a useful guide (Fig. 5.11).

5.1.2.2 Lymphoma

Except when node biopsy is indicated to establish the etiology of a lesion, node dissection is never justified simply to determine whether or

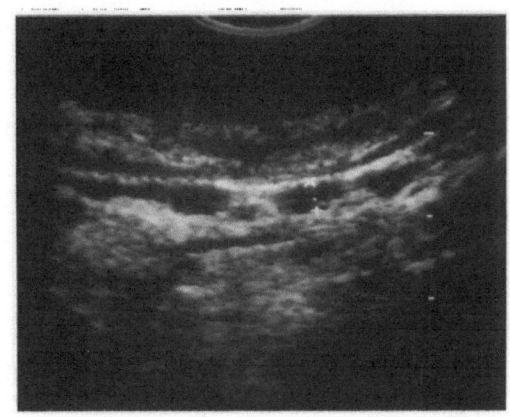

Fig. 5.6. Small inflammatory nodes caused by subcutaneous cellulitis (3 mm between the two *crosses*)

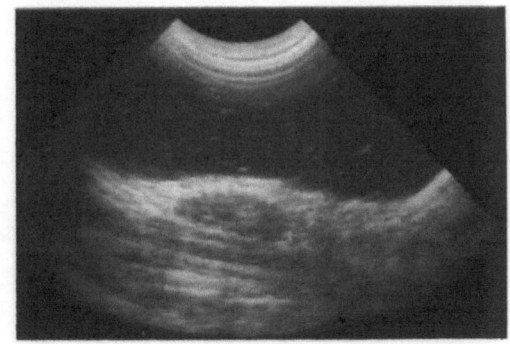

Fig. 5.7. Small inflammatory spinal chain node (transverse diameter 5 mm)

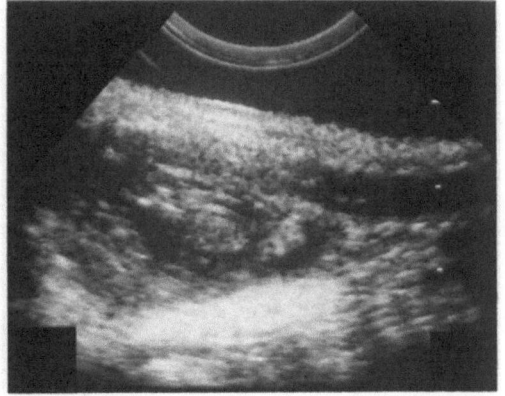

Fig. 5.8. Large inflammatory node resulting from an oral abscess

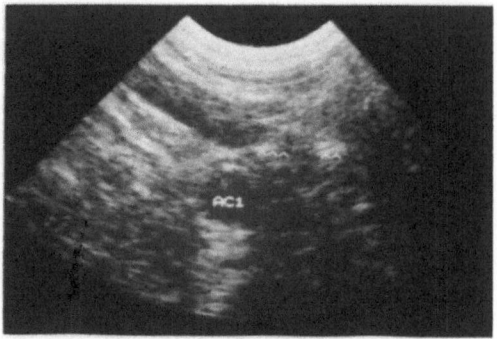

Fig. 5.9. Small postirradiation nodal calcifications *(arrows)* with acoustic shadows. *AC1,* common carotid artery

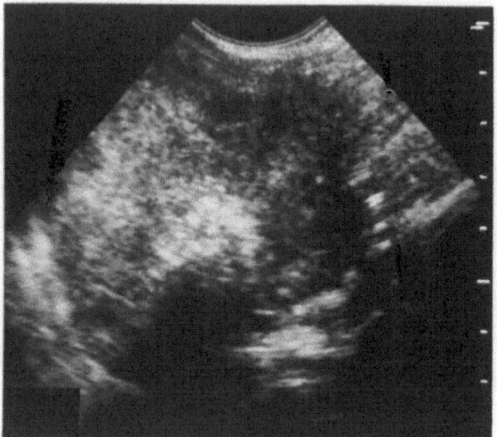

Fig. 5.10. Central calcification in a large cervical node after radiotherapy

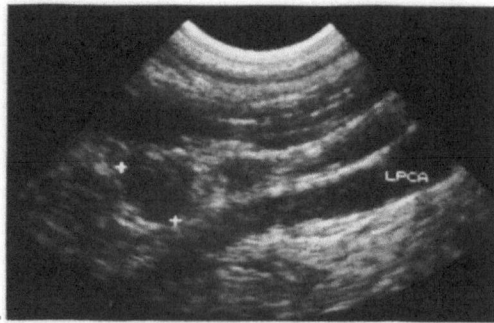

Fig. 5.11. Subclinical metastatic node (11 mm between the two *crosses*). *LPCA,* left common carotid artery

not a lymphoma has spread to the neck. Consequently, no anatomic correlations have ever been published in the literature. Particular care must thus be taken to avoid false positive errors. We therefore do not consider multiple enlarged nodes indicative of lymphoma unless at least one of the nodes has a transverse diameter of 10 mm or more. US-directed aspiration biopsy is indicated whenever doubt persists.

5.1.2.3 Inflammatory Nodes

Most, but not all, inflammatory nodes are smaller than 8 mm in diameter. The infectious process (abscess, cellulitis) and pain that habitually accompany larger nodes suffice to suggest the diagnosis, thereby obviating the need for US-directed node biopsy.

5.1.3 Vascular Relations

Accurate evaluation of the relations between nodes and the internal jugular vein is particularly important, especially for enlarged jugulocarotid nodes. A Valsalva maneuver may be necessary for satisfactory examination. As a reminder, the internal jugular veins are not necessarily symmetrical. Large nodal masses such as metastatic nodes can displace or even invade and thrombose the internal jugular vein. By contrast, in our experience, not even large lymphomatous nodes cause jugular vein thrombosis. Until such time as the obligatory anatomic proof is obtained, a nodal mass larger than 7 cm adjacent to the jugulocarotid vessels can be considered metastatic if it causes jugular vein thrombosis, and lymphomatous if the jugular vein coursing through the nodal group is intact (Figs. 5.12–5.17). Inflammatory pathologies do not cause jugular vein thrombosis unless an endoluminal venous process is responsible for inflammation of the lateral neck. The carotid artery may be displaced, but actual vascular invasion by metastatic nodes does not occur until late in the course of the disease (Figs. 5.18 and 5.19).

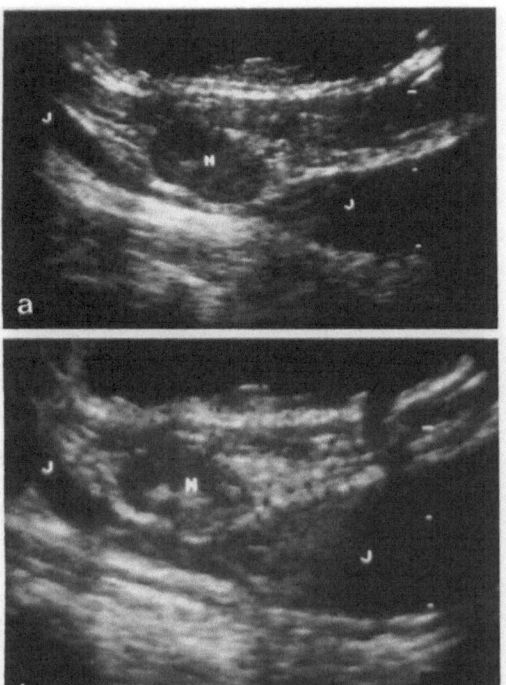

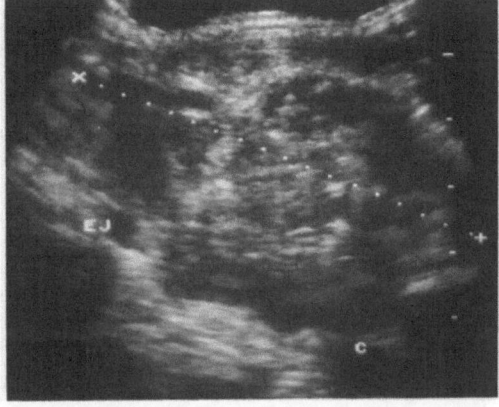

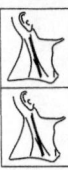

Fig. 5.12 a, b. Relations of a metastatic node *(N)* with the internal jugular vein. **a** Image in apnea showing severe compression or thrombosis of the internal jugular vein. *(J)* **b** Severe compression of the nonthrombosed internal jugular vein *(J)* is evident after a Valsalva maneuver

Fig. 5.14. Thrombosis of the internal jugular vein by a large metastatic node, accompanied by dilatation of the external jugular vein *(EJ)* and posterior displacement (but no invasion) of the carotid artery *(C)*

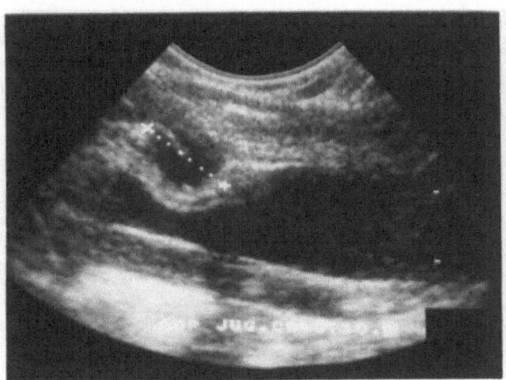

Fig. 5.13. Compression of the internal jugular vein by an enlarged node (14 mm between the two *crosses*)

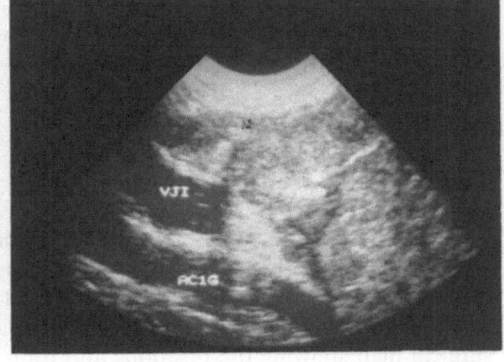

Fig. 5.15. Complete thrombosis of the internal jugular vein *(VJI)* by a large metastatic node *(ADP)*. The left common carotid artery *(ACIG)* is merely displaced

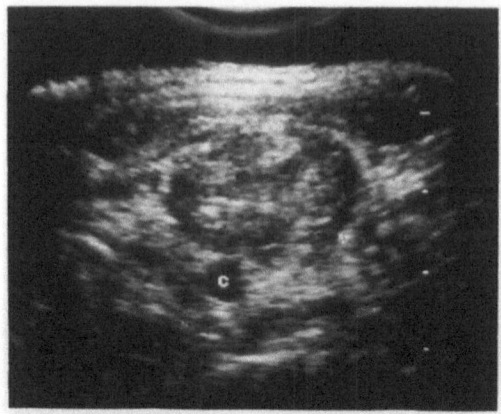

Fig. 5.16. Thrombosis of the internal jugular vein anterior to the common carotid artery *(C)*

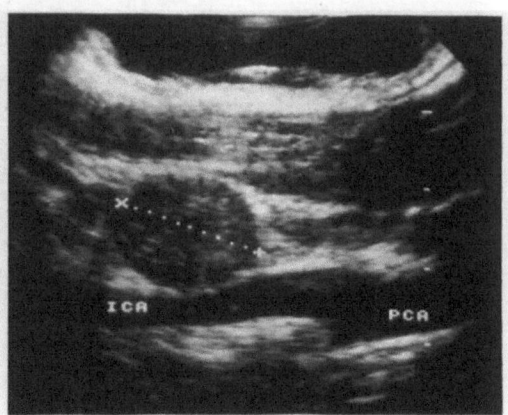

Fig. 5.18. Discrete displacement of the internal carotid artery *(ICA)* by a metastatic node. *PCA*, common carotid artery (20 mm between the two *crosses*)

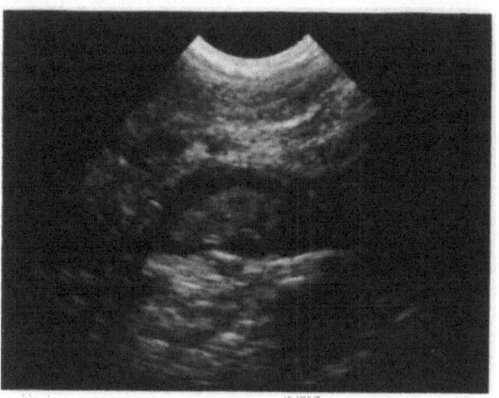

Fig. 5.17. Lower limit of a jugular vein thrombus caused by invasion of the suprajacent internal jugular vein by a large nodal mass

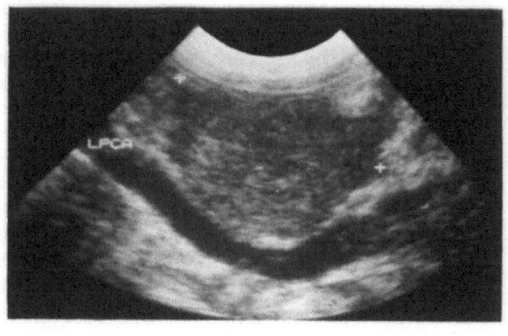

Fig. 5.19. Considerable displacement of the left common carotid artery *(LPCA)* by a metastatic node (31 mm between the two *crosses*); no vascular invasion

5.1.4 *Presentation of Results*

Clear presentation of sonographic findings for the nonspecialist physician is of prime importance. Transfer of information can be facilitated if, along with the usual sonogram report, a surgical map showing the positions and transverse diameters of nodes and their relations with the internal jugular vein is prepared. Division of such charts into eight cervical regions allows easy evaluation of results. Carotid artery involvement by ENT cancer must be an extremely rare finding during pretherapy work-

ups, and we ourselves have never even encountered invasion of the adventitia during staging examinations (cf. Chap. 1).

5.1.5 *Differential Diagnosis*

The differential diagnosis of enlarged cervical nodes depends on whether only one or several lesions are present.

5.1.5.1 Multiple Lesions

Multinodular lesions involve no diagnostic problems. The major difficulty is obtainment of accurate topographic data rather than identification of such masses as enlarged nodes.

5.1.5.2 Solitary Lesions

The possibility that a solitary, nonthyroid, nonsalivary, nonvascular cervical mass is an enlarged lymph node can only be suggested if there is a neoplastic or lymphomatous context. From a purely sonographic standpoint, an anechogenic nodule in the midjugulocarotid region, along the anterior belly of the sternocleidomastoid muscle, may be a branchial or lymphoepithelial cyst. By contrast, thyroglossal duct cysts usually occupy a midline infrahyoid or prehyoid position (cf. Chap. 6). Vascular tumefaction (aneurysm, phlebectasia) is readily identified by US. Solid solitary nodules may have a rare etiology such as a neurogenic tumor. Solitary sarcomatous lesions tend to be larger in diameter than nodal lesions.

5.2 Nonultrasonographic Techniques for Cervical Node Examination

5.2.1 Cervical Lymphography

The opacification procedure used in cervical lymphography, the longest established technique for examination of the cervical nodes, is similar to that employed for the lower limbs. Catheterization is not always easy, but there are no complications owing to the small amount of contrast material used. The lymphographic features of neck lesions are comparable to those of lower limb pathologies, especially for lymphomatous and metastatic processes. There are no longer any indications for this technique, which always required associated cervical node dissection for patients with ENT cancer. In like manner, the information provided by lymphoscintigraphy (Senda and Sasaki 1980) has not proved sufficiently determinant to warrant systematic use of this technique for cervical node pathologies.

5.2.2 Carotid Angiography

Carotid angiography can diagnose vascular compression and invasion by a large cervical nodal mass, and was formerly used preoperatively when vascular involvement that would have prevented complete surgical exeresis of a tumor was suspected. Arterial infiltration was rarely observed although large masses often caused venous thrombosis (especially of the internal jugular vein). Angiograms obtained after carotid opacification showed flow derivation during the venous return phase.

Carotid angiography is performed with the patient under local anesthesia using new contrast materials which cause no pain when injected. Despite the possibilities offered by arterial digital subtraction angiography, carotid angiography is currently of little interest owing to the high sensitivity of US for identification of jugular vein thrombosis secondary to compression by a nodal mass.

5.2.3 Computed Tomography

CT is of unquestionable value for cervical node explorations as it can determine both the number and position of enlarged nodes and their relations with the neck vessels. However, an intravenous contrast material must be used for analysis of vascular relations. Like US, CT can visualize lesions but not differentiate between inflammatory and tumoral etiologies. In addition, CT is unable to demonstrate extracapsular extension for small nodal lesions. CT thus has the same limitations as US for lymph node studies. By contrast, CT allows thorough topographic investigations of ENT tumors, including searches for nodal metastases, and especially those in retropharyngeal sites (Mancuso et al. 1981). CT is also indicated for detection of the subclinical lymphomatous lesions frequently found in Waldeyer's ring.

5.3 Ultrasonography of Metastatic Nodes of ENT Cancer

Numerous studies have emphasized the failure of physical examination to detect lymph node metastases in patients with ENT cancer. Depending on the series the incidence of false negative errors varies from 27.6% to 38.1%. Moreover, when a nodal mass in the lateral neck occurs concomitantly with a primary ENT tumor, physical examination cannot determine whether or not the jugular vein is truly thrombosed. Of the various imaging techniques described in Sect. 5.2, only CT is of major interest for nodal studies as it is the sole procedure, apart from magnetic resonance imaging, capable of detecting deep metastatic nodes.

5.3.1 Node Size

In patients with a recognized ENT tumor, all nodes with a transverse diameter over 8 mm are considered metastatic. These nodes are generally solid, and care must be taken to analyze their exact relations with the jugular vein. In a prospective study of 100 patients, we demonstrated the superiority of real-time, high-frequency ultrasound over physical examination; comparison of US and anatomic data revealed a sensitivity of 92.6% for US vs 78% for physical examination. Physical examination had a specificity of 97% vs 91% for US. US identified all 18 cases of internal jugular vein thrombosis whereas physical examination suggested this situation for only 5 patients. US examination modified the clinical staging in 28% of the cases in this series (Bruneton et al. 1984). These results, which have been confirmed by other investigations (Hajek et al. 1984), highlight the effectiveness of US, which can often change the therapeutic strategy.

The selection of 8 mm as the cutoff point for definition of metastatic nodes of ENT cancers obviously results in some false positive errors corresponding to inflammatory nodes (Fig. 5.20), but, as shown in our series, the incidence of such errors is low. In the same manner, nodes smaller than 8 mm may be ENT cancer metastases. Nevertheless, use of this statistically determined threshold value reduces the percentages of both false negative and false positive errors for metastatic nodes to a minimum.

5.3.2 Ultrasonography and Pretherapy Workup of Metastatic Nodes

Pretherapy workups must obviously determine whether there is any venous thrombosis and/or bilateral nodal involvement. Jugular vein thrombosis precludes a modified neck dissection; in addition to node exeresis, the mandatory radical procedure involves removal of the internal jugular vein, the spinal nerve, and the sternocleidomastoid muscle. The value of US for the workup of superficial nodes during ENT cancers is heightened by its topographic accuracy.

5.3.2.1 Detection of Subclinical Homolateral Nodes

More sensitive than physical examination, ultrasound allows the detection of small subclinical homolateral nodes. This is especially true for patients with thick necks.

5.3.2.2 Accurate Analysis of the Size of Palpable Nodes

As US can accurately determine lesion size, the sonogram constitutes an invaluable reference document for the surveillance of patients treated nonsurgically. This is increasingly the case owing to the present trend toward the use of induction (neoadjuvant) chemotherapy. Precise volumetric data on superficial nodes is ex-

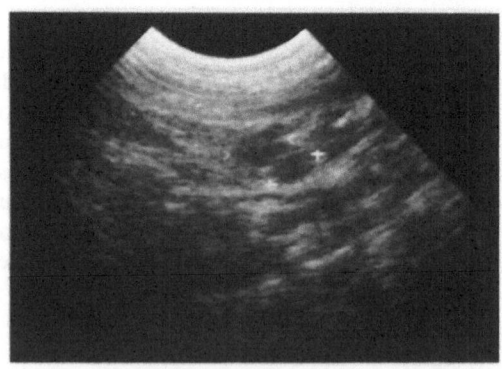

Fig. 5.20. Small metastatic nodes (7 mm between the two *crosses*) from a carcinoma of the external auditory canal. This was a case of false negative error with US, because images were misinterpreted as inflammatory nodes

tremely helpful for monitoring response to therapy in such cases. By contrast, neither US nor any other imaging technique can currently detect extracapsular extension for lesions smaller than 1 cm in transverse diameter.

5.3.2.3 Analysis of Vascular Relations

As mentioned earlier, US is sufficiently sensitive to detect thrombosis. The only potential pitfall to avoid with internal jugular vein thrombosis is confusion of a dilated anterior, posterior, or external jugular vein with a markedly displaced internal jugular vein.

5.3.2.4 Analysis of the Contralateral Cervical Node Regions

Disease spread to the contralateral neck is not uncommon, and modifies the therapeutic protocol. Pathological contralateral nodes are usually small, and the discrepancy between the sensitivity of US and that of physical examination is at a maximum in these cases.

5.3.3 Ultrasonography and Monitoring of Nonsurgical Treatment

Along with its determinant role in the staging of ENT cancers, US is an ideal method for monitoring the course of patients who do not undergo surgery. Being less invasive than CT, ultrasonography is particularly indicated for follow-up studies aimed at assessing the efficacy of chemotherapy or radiotherapy. This is especially true for patients with radiation-induced cutaneous thickening of the neck. Even though a primary ENT tumor may be well controlled, the prognosis often depends on the status of the cervical nodes (Bartelink et al. 1982; Jesse and Fletcher 1963; Mustard and Rosen 1963). Our analysis of patients followed up for cervical node involvement which was not treated by surgery confirmed these classical data. Of the 33 patients for whom sonograms demonstrated stable or progressive disease, only 2 were still alive at 1 year. By contrast, only 9 of 67 patients with a sonographically demonstrated improvement in node status died in less

than 12 months (Bruneton et al. 1984). These findings emphasize the importance of regular, effective monitoring of node size during therapy. Whereas chemotherapy does not alter the nature of the skin of the neck, irradiation generally causes cutaneous thickening which reduces the value of physical examination even further. Even though its sensitivity remains markedly superior to that of physical examination, US can also be hampered by postirradiation induration (Figs. 5.21 and 5.22). In our experience CT is more sensitive than US in such cases, whereas the opposite is true for pretherapy workups.

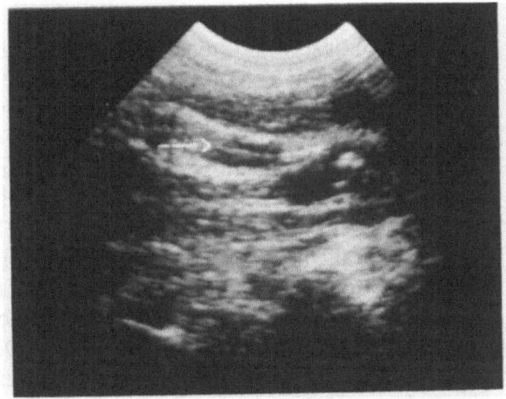

Fig. 5.21. Residual nodal tissue after irradiation

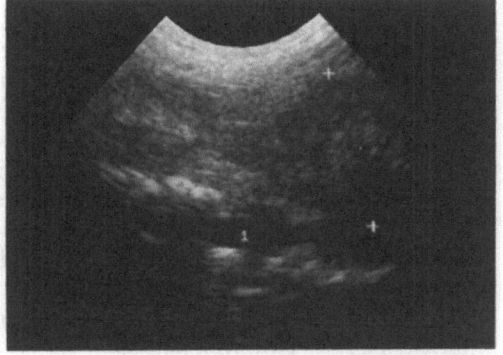

Fig. 5.22. Cervical node recurrence after radiotherapy. The mass was hard to palpate because of its moderate size and postirradiation skin thickening (19 mm between the two *crosses*). *1*, right common carotid artery

We currently perform US systematically as part of the pretherapy nodal workup for ENT cancer patients; CT is utilized for tumor staging and searches for deep-seated metastatic nodes. CT appears of greatest value in patients who have been treated by radiotherapy, as US seems less sensitive in these cases. Nevertheless, US remains the basic technique for the surveillance of treated nodal disease. Thanks to widespread use of US, the clinical N stage of the TNM classification will undoubtedly be replaced by a sonographic N in the future.

5.4 Ultrasonography of Lymphomatous Cervical Nodes

Non-Hodgkin's lymphoma (NHL) nodes are usually hypoechogenic, and may even have a pseudocystic appearance. Such patterns are rare with Hodgkin's disease (HD) nodes, which tend to be solid. Generally speaking, the clinical importance of US studies differs for HD and for NHL because the prognosis for NHL depends on the histologic type, whereas in HD it tends to depend on the disease site(s). The sensitivity required for detection of subclinical nodal involvement therefore also differs. Discovery of a subclinical lymphomatous inguinal node in an HD patient reflects subdiaphragmatic disease spread and thus a less favorable outcome. By contrast, the implications of one or more involved inguinal nodes are less serious for NHL patients; such nodes merely constitute additional targets requiring surveillance during treatment.

Physical examination of lymphomatous cervical nodes can be difficult. As opposed to metastatic nodes, which feel firm or even hard, lymphomatous nodes are often soft. Physical examination will therefore not be positive unless the lymphomatous node is relatively large or there are several involved nodes (Fierstein and Thawley 1978; MacNelis and Pai 1969).

Node consistency is not a source of difficulty for US analysis. However, particular care is required for evaluation of the spinal chain, which is not always systematically examined for certain ENT cancers. Palpable lesions, and particularly those in the spinal region, may not be visualized unless US is performed with a water bath or Reston interface. Analysis of the cervical regions of patients with lymphoma should thus be performed both before and after installation of a water bath or Reston interface coupled with a 7.5 or 10 MHz transducer (Figs. 5.23 and 5.24).

Whereas the value of clinical, ultrasound, and surgical findings can be compared for the workup and surveillance of ENT cancers, and particularly cervical node involvement, this is not possible for superficial lymphomatous nodes which have no surgical indication. Nevertheless, identification of a node or nodes with a minimum transverse diameter of 10 mm together with the presence of multiple nodal lesions generally suggests lymphoma. Comparison of

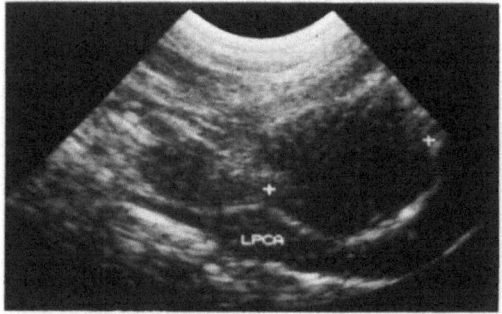

Fig. 5.23. Hodgkin's disease nodes lateral to the carotid artery. *LPCA*, left common carotid artery. (24 mm between the two *crosses*)

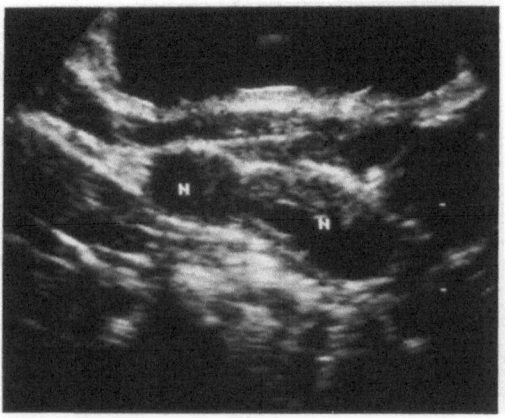

Fig. 5.24. Spinal chain nodes *(N)* in a patient with Hodgkin's disease

clinical and US findings for the cervical and supraclavicular regions reveals that US can detect 17.7% of the nodal sites (both HD and NHL) missed clinically. Likewise, during patient follow-up, US visualized lesions undetected by physical examination in 15.8% of patients who developed cervical node recurrence. In the absence of other disease sites indicative of progressive disease, US-directed node biopsy is indicated for selection of the most appropriate therapeutic approach (Bruneton et al. 1985). It is our policy to systematically examine the superficial node regions (cervical nodes, axillary nodes using a transpectoral approach, inguinal nodes) of all lymphoma patients for both staging and follow-up purposes.

5.5 Inflammatory Disease

Ultrasonography is relatively less helpful for the investigation of inflammatory disease than for ENT tumors and lymphomas. Inflammatory nodes tend to be small, although an abscess or cellulitis can cause considerable node enlargement (over 20 mm in transverse diameter). Node size generally reflects the severity of the inflammation. Widespread administration of antibiotics and anti-inflammatory drugs at an early stage means that the neck is rarely examined sonographically in these cases, and inflammation rarely attains severe proportions. Head and neck infections susceptible to cause nodal enlargement greater than 20 mm in transverse diameter are more common in immunocompromised patients. Tuberculosis can also cause enlargement of multiple cervical nodes, but the etiological diagnosis cannot be determined by US alone.

5.6 Conclusion

Ultrasonography is particularly indicated for the investigation of cervical node pathologies. As there are many benefits provided by real-time apparatus and high frequency transducers, US should be a routine part of all cervical studies. For example, thyroid cancer can be suspected after cervical US if even a small nodule is associated with at least one homolateral nodal mass. The same holds true for salivary gland tumors.

Ultrasonography currently appears to be a sufficiently reliable technique for gauging ENT cancers so that the clinical N stage of the TNM classification could be replaced by an ultrasonographic N. US exploration of the superficial lymph node-bearing regions, including the neck, also appears indispensable for the staging and follow-up of lymphoma patients. When US findings are normal, examination can be completed in less than 10 min.

The undeniable value of ultrasonography of the superficial nodes is, however, moderated by two factors. Firstly, as the resolution of sonograms allows detection of subclinical lesions, more widespread availability of transducers suited for US guidance of node biopsies is desirable. Secondly, our personal results were obtained after a period of mandatory examiner training which, like familiarity with abdominal ultrasound, is indispensable to obtain the maximum benefits from US.

5.7 References

Bartelink H, Breur K, Hart G (1982) Radiotherapy of lymph node metastases in patients with squamous cell carcinoma of the head and neck region. Int J Radiat Oncol Biol Phys 8: 983–989

Bruneton JN, Roux P, Caramella E, Demard F, Vallicioni J, Chauvel P (1984) Ear, nose and throat cancer: ultrasound diagnosis of metastasis to cervical lymph nodes. Radiology 152: 771–773

Bruneton JN, Caramella E, Manzino JJ, Fenart D, Occelli JP, Balu-Maestro C (1985) Ultrasound examination of superficial lymph nodes in lymphomas. J Ultrasound Med 4: 11

Fierstein JT, Thawley SE (1978) Lymphoma of the head and neck. Laryngoscope 88: 582–593

Hajek PC, Tuerk R, Czembirek H, Tscholakoff D, Kumpan W, Salomonswitz E (1984) Assessment of cervical lymph node pathology by ultrasound: a clinical study. Radiology 153 (P): 82

Jesse RH, Fletcher GH (1963) Metastases in cervical lymph nodes from oropharyngeal carcinoma: treatments and results. AJR 90: 990–996

MacGavran MH, Bauer WC, Ogura JH (1961) The incidence of cervical lymph node metastases from epidermoid carcinoma of the larynx and their relationship to certain characteristics of the primary tumor. A study based on the clinical and pathological findings for 96 patients treated by primary en bloc laryngectomy and radical neck dissection. Cancer 14: 55–66

MacNelis FL, Pai VT (1969) Malignant lymphoma of head and neck. Laryngoscope 79: 1076–1087

Mancuso AA, Maceri D, Rice DH, Hanafee W (1981) CT of cervical lymph node cancer. Radiology 136: 381-385

Manfredi D, Jacobelli G (1975) Neck dissection in the treatment of head and neck cancer: results in 1162 cases. In: Chambers RG, Janssen de Limpens AMP, Jaques DA, Routledge RT (eds) Cancer of the head and neck. Excerpta Medica, Amsterdam, pp 221-224

Martis C, Karabouta I, Lazaridis N (1979) Incidence of lymph node metastasis in elective (prophylactic) neck dissection for oral carcinoma. J Maxillofac Surg 7: 182-191

Mountford RA, Atkinson P (1979) Doppler ultrasound examination of pathologically enlarged lymph nodes. Br J Radiol 52: 464-467

Mustard RA, Rosen IB (1963) Cervical lymph node involvement in oral cancer. AJR 90: 978-989

Sako K, Pradier RN, Marchetta FC, Pickren JW (1964) Fallibility of palpation in the diagnosis of metastases to cervical nodes. Surg Gynecol Obstet 118: 989-990

Senda K, Sasaki T (1980) Scintigram of the cervical lymph nodes. Rinsho Hoshasen 25: 413-414

6 Other Cervical Sites

J.-N. BRUNETON AND D. FENART

Ultrasound (US) studies are currently of limited value for all of the pathologies and structures dealt with in this chapter. In addition to oral cavity pathologies, neurogenic tumors, cervical cysts, and cases of local regional spread of cancer to the neck, there are several rare etiologies for which the US pattern is only one of several diagnostic factors or merely confirms the clinical diagnosis. There are also certain US applications whose value has only been recognized rather recently (staging of oral lesions, analysis of speech and the oral phase of swallowing).

6.1 Oral Cavity

Tumors in the lower part of the oral cavity can be visualized by ultrasonography performed using a submental approach. US imaging capabilities are limited by structure size, but local tumor extension can often be analyzed satisfactorily. As demonstrated by Shawker et al. (1985), US is also an excellent technique for analysis of speech disorders and the oral phase of swallowing.

6.1.1 Cancer of the Tongue

Cancer of the tongue is one of the most common malignancies of the upper aerodigestive tract. The prognosis is poor, especially if nodal involvement is already evident at initial presentation.

6.1.1.1 General Features

Pathologically, most oral lesions correspond to squamous cell carcinoma, 5%-10% of which develop from preexisting mucosal lesions (leukoplakia, exophytic keratosis, lichen planus, chronic glossitis). The majority of squamous cell carcinomas of the tongue are of the ulcerating-infiltrative type, and nodal metastases are frequent. Other types of malignant tumors, accounting for scarcely 2% of all lingual tumors, include glandular tumors (cylindroma), mesenchymal sarcomas, and especially lymphomas (the sites of predilection being the base of the tongue and the lingual tonsil). Secondary tumors of the tongue are extremely rare. Cancers of the tongue represent approximately 20% of all cancers of the upper aerodigestive tract. In France, they account for around 1% of all cancers; the incidence is similar in most Western countries (Whitaker et al. 1972).

The mean age of patients with lingual carcinomas is the same as that for squamous cell carcinomas of the upper aerodigestive tract, between 50 and 70 years. Male predominance is especially marked in France. A similar male predominance exists in other countries for cancers of the base of the tongue. By contrast, for cancers of the mobile or oral tongue (anterior two-thirds), the former male: female ratio of 2:1 in the United States of America has changed considerably in the past 2 decades due to a steady rise in the number of females affected. The two major *predisposing factors* are chronic use of tobacco and alcohol. Chronic oral and dental infections undoubtedly play an important etiological role.

Topographically, squamous cell carcinomas of the tongue can be divided into lesions affecting the oral tongue and those occurring at the base of the tongue. The circumvallate papillae are usually used as the dividing line between these two parts. Approximately one-third of cancers affect the base of the tongue; two-thirds affect the oral tongue. Cancers occurring at the junction between these two parts involve problems for classification; they account for 5%-10% of all lingual cancers and are generally studied with cancers of the mobile tongue. The site of predilection on the mobile tongue is the lateral borders.

6.1.1.2 Squamous Cell Carcinoma of the Oral Tongue

The most frequent presenting symptoms are irritation and pain; patients with advanced lesions may complain of ear pain. Discovery of a cervical nodal mass by the patient is a less frequent reason for diagnosis. Physical examination usually detects an ulcerating-infiltrative tumor. Digital palpation must be performed systematically to evaluate:

- medial extension towards the midline
- lateral and anterior extension towards the floor of the mouth, the gums, and the mandible
- posterior extension towards the base of the tongue, the anterior tonsillar pillar, and the tonsillar fossa

Ultrasound evaluation of tumoral spread is performed in the same manner, using a submental approach. Findings obtained by physical and US examination serve as the basis for the T category of the TNM classification:

Tis   preinvasive carcinoma in situ
T1   greatest diameter of primary tumor 2 cm or less
T2   greatest diameter of primary tumor more than 2 cm but not more than 4 cm
T3   greatest diameter of primary tumor more than 4 cm

Nodal involvement is already clinically evident in 40%–60% of patients at the time of initial presentation; 10%–15% of patients have bilateral lesions (Vandenbrouck et al. 1970). The site of predilection is the submaxillary region, followed by spread to the jugular chain nodes.
Depending on equipment availability, staff policy, and the stage of the disease, the therapeutic alternatives for primary tumors and metastatic nodes include surgery, radiotherapy, and chemotherapy. Survival at 5 years varies with the stage and whether there is any nodal involvement, but can generally be estimated at

60% (Decroix and Ghossein 1981; Frazell and Lucas 1962; Pierquin et al. 1970; Vermund et al. 1984).

6.1.1.3 Squamous Cell Carcinoma of the Base of the Tongue

Presenting symptoms are often of late onset and rarely suggest the diagnosis; they include moderate pain, a foreign body sensation, and, in one-third of cases, an enlarged cervical node. After indirect mirror examination, palpation is essential to assess:

- anterior extension towards the oral tongue
- posterior extension towards the vallecula epiglottica and the suprahyoid epiglottis
- lateral extension along the glossotonsillar sulcus, the tonsil and its pillars, and the pharyngoepiglottic fold

Ultrasonography performed using a submental approach allows similar analyses. The TNM classification used for the oral tongue also applies to cancers of the tongue base. Searches for cervical node involvement essentially concern the jugular chain nodes.
Primary tumors of the tongue base are usually treated by radiotherapy, alone or in combination with surgery or chemotherapy. Regardless of the therapeutic approach, the 5-year prognosis has not been significantly improved during the last 2 decades, and still stands at an average of 20% at 5 years (Strong 1979; Vermund et al. 1984).

6.1.1.4 Other Malignant Tumors of the Tongue

Lymphomas of the tongue base or the lingual tonsil are the least frequent sites of lymphomatous involvement of Waldeyer's ring. The prognosis for these usually large masses is better than that for squamous cell carcinomas of the tongue base (Bruneton et al. 1986b).
Salivary gland tumors, and especially cylindromas, tend to affect the base of the tongue; these lesions usually grow slowly but are apt to recur locally.

6.1.1.5 Nonultrasonographic Imaging of Lingual Cancers

As demonstrated by Apter et al. (1984), lateral soft-tissue radiographs of the neck can identify relatively large exophytic lesions at the level of the tongue base. These authors also pointed out the value of exploring the tongue base area using double contrast radiography of the pharynx. Use of a high density barium suspension permits visualization of small tongue base tumors immediately after the dynamic examination.

Neither these simple radiological techniques nor CT are sufficient for satisfactory staging of small oral tongue tumors, although CT allows acceptable analysis of tongue base cancers. For Larsson et al. (1982), CT has an excellent sensitivity (28 out of 30 patients staged correctly) for evaluating the relations of both tongue base and floor of the mouth lesions with the midline. However, dental fillings can affect the quality of both transverse and coronal CT scans.

6.1.1.6 Ultrasonography of Lingual Cancers

Being noninvasive, ultrasonography is easy to perform. Moreover, movement of the transducer over the submental area is generally painless, as opposed to intraoral digital palpation which many patients find hard to tolerate.

Sonographically, lingual tumors present as a mass of decreased echogenicity relative to the normal adjacent musculature. Although small lesions may appear homogeneous, the complex internal structure is readily demonstrated once tumors attain 2 cm in greatest dimension. Ulcerations of at least 5 mm can be visualized if they contain air or serous fluids. Particular care is required when determining tumoral margins; this may be no problem for T2 tumors, but can be difficult for certain large, locally invasive lesions (Figs. 6.1–6.3). Midline, lateral, and anterior-posterior tumoral extension (cf. Sect. 5. 6.1.1.2 and 6.1.1.3) must be evaluated sonographically using the technique described in Chap. 1. Ultrasonography has an excellent sensitivity for demonstrating tumoral spread towards the midline and extension to deep structures. By contrast, US has several obvious topographical limitations. The shortcomings of

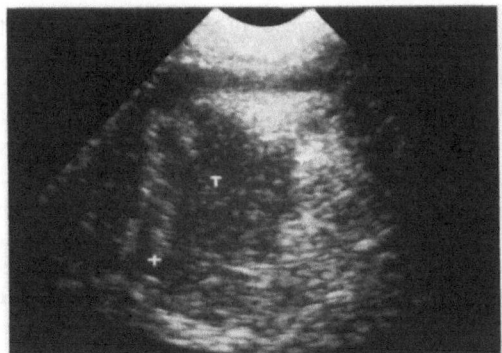

Fig. 6.1. Cancer of the base of the tongue (37 mm in diameter); only the deep portion of the tumor crosses the midline slightly

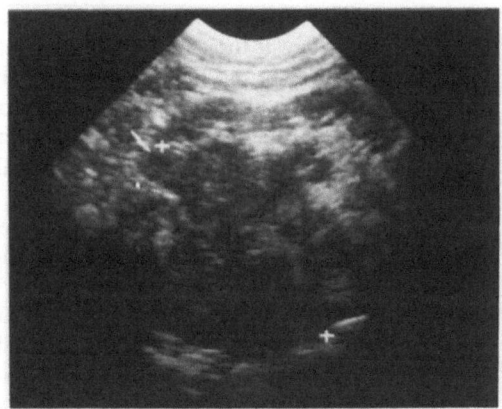

Fig. 6.2. Large tumor invading almost the entire tongue (45 mm between the two *crosses*)

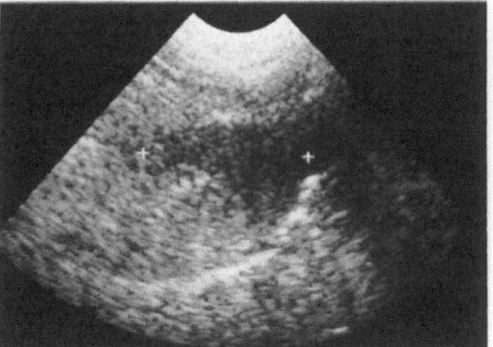

Fig. 6.3. Cancer of the base of the tongue (37 mm between the two *crosses*)

US studies are especially evident for cancer of the oral tongue. No imaging technique is really satisfactory for analysis of this site, however, and physical examination is certainly the most accurate procedure for staging purposes. This situation is understandable because the oral tongue lies free within the oral cavity, and patients often find it hard to keep their tongue in the low position required for satisfactory US examination by a submental approach. Small tumors on the lateral borders of the oral tongue are also occasionally hard to evaluate by US.

Problems related to lesion size include small T1 tumors, which are not always visible with US and correspond to shallow infiltration (less than 1 cm deep). Likewise, although bulky tumors which may have spread towards the mandible can be seen on sonograms, the transducer's field of view is too small to obtain a satisfactory global view, and CT is preferable. By contrast, the sensitivity and innocuousness of US makes it an excellent technique for examining the base of the tongue (Bruneton et al. 1986 b).

The existence of metastatic cervical nodes modifies both the surgical approach and the prognosis (cf. Chap. 5). The frequency of nodal involvement makes thorough exploration of the lymph node-bearing regions of the neck particularly important. Workup of oral tongue lesions requires that particular care be paid to the submaxillary areas; for tongue base cancers, attention must be concentrated on the jugular chain nodes, because nodal involvement in this region conditions both the therapeutic attitude and the prognosis.

Ultrasonography is generally not very satisfactory for the follow-up of treated patients. While searches for metastatic cervical nodes are always worthwhile, US detection of local disease recurrence is generally difficult. After partial glossectomy, for example, the greater volume of air surrounding the remaining portion of the tongue in the oral cavity precludes acceptable evaluation. If no preirradiation document is available for reference use, it may prove impossible after radiotherapy to tell whether a hypoechogenic image is a postirradiation sequel or corresponds to local disease recurrence. Finally, the limitations of US for pre- and posttherapy nodal explorations have been indicated in Chap. 5.

Overall, ultrasonography is indicated for the exploration of T2 and T3 tumors of the tongue; it is also particularly helpful for evaluation of tongue base lesions. Regardless of the site or stage of the disease, US is indispensable for the workup of lingual cancers.

6.1.2 Cancer of the Floor of the Mouth

Less frequent than lingual carcinoma, cancer of the floor of the mouth represents approximately 10% of all upper aerodigestive tract malignancies. There is a marked male predominance; mean patient age is between 50 and 70 years and, as for cancers of the tongue, chronic alcoholism and tobacco use are predisposing factors. As a reminder, the floor of the mouth is the U-shaped space bounded by the inferior surface of the oral tongue and the medial surface of the lower gum. The floor of the mouth is supported by the mylohyoid muscle.

Pathologically, almost all tumors of the floor of the mouth are squamous cell carcinomas; they usually manifest as an ulceration, which is frequently hidden by the tongue. Tumoral spread occurs both superficially and towards deep structures, along the submandibular gland duct and the sublingual glands, into the lingual musculature, and thence into the submaxillary space. Tumor extension is also possible towards the pelvilingual sulcus and the tongue. Nearly two-thirds of patients already have clinically positive nodes at first presentation; whether involved uni- or bilaterally, the submaxillary nodes are affected most often, followed by the jugular chain nodes. Cancers of the floor of the mouth have a particularly poor prognosis; regardless of the therapeutic approach, the survival rate at 5 years is only 30% (Dulac et al. 1975; Pierquin et al. 1970; Richard et al. 1975).

CT allows satisfactory exploration of the floor of the mouth, especially if coronal sections can be obtained. It is the imaging procedure of choice for large tumors, both for evaluation of soft tissue involvement and detection of concomitant bone lesions. Moderately sized lesions no greater than 4 cm in length can be analyzed by ultrasonography; along with evaluating spread to deep structures, US can detect

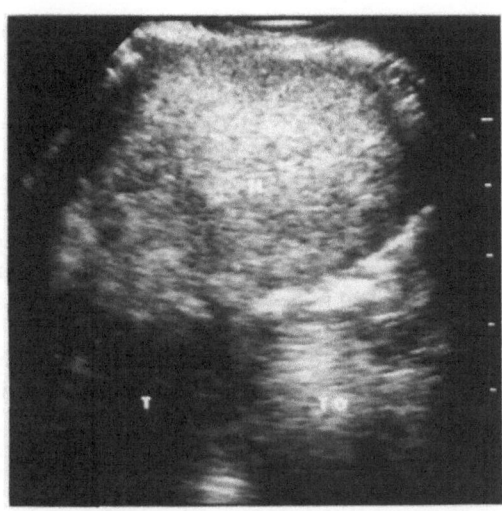

 Fig. 6.4. Tumor of the floor of the mouth *(T)* displacing the tongue *(TO)* towards the opposite side, complicated by a large submaxillary nodal mass *(N)*

metastatic nodes, which are apt to be bilateral. The limitations of ultrasonography for cancers of the floor of the mouth are essentially topographic in nature; tumors smaller than 1 cm in diameter are usually very shallow, and may not be visible on sonograms. A large tumor that has spread to bone is an indication for CT rather than US, at least for evaluation of the tumor itself (Fig. 6.4).

6.1.3 Cancer of the Tonsil

Ultrasonography using an external approach does not allow analysis of cancers of the soft palate, which certain authors group together with tonsillar neoplasia. Only cancers of the tonsillar region can be investigated by US, and these are the sole lesions dealt with in this section. As a reminder, the originality of the tonsil resides in its lymphoepithelial makeup (malpighian epithelium plus lymphoid tissue).

6.1.3.1 General Features

Pathologically, most cancers of the tonsil are epitheliomas, usually squamous cell carcinomas. Lymphoepithelioma is the result of simultaneous malignant change of the epithelial and lymphoid tissues of the tonsil. After epitheliomas, malignant lymphomas represent the second most frequent cause of tonsillar cancer. Involvement of the cervical nodes is common with both epitheliomas and lymphomas.

Cancer of the tonsil is less frequent than cancer of the tongue but more so than cancer of the floor of the mouth; tonsillar malignancies represent approximately 1% of all cancers. Squamous cell carcinomas account for 85%–95% of tonsillar neoplasia; the incidence of lymphoma varies from 5%–15% (Terz and Farr 1967).

The mean age of patients with squamous cell tonsillar cancer ranges from 50 to 70 years; as for other squamous cell carcinomas of the oral cavity, there is a marked male predominance. Chronic alcoholism and abuse of tobacco are well-known predisposing factors. The age range for malignant tonsillar lymphomas is much wider, and their frequency in males is only slightly higher than in females.

6.1.3.2 Squamous Cell Carcinoma of the Tonsil

The most common presenting symptom is unilateral dysphagia, occasionally accompanied by ear pain. At initial presentation one-third of patients have a cervical neck mass; often, this is the sign that has motivated the patient to consult a physician.

The gross appearance of a tonsillar tumor can generally be described as a growth, ulceration, invasion, or as a combination of these forms. Investigation of tumoral extension requires systematic evaluation of:

- medial spread towards the base of the tongue, and the area of the lingual junction
- posterior spread towards the lateral pharyngeal wall
- superomedial spread onto the soft palate
- anterolateral spread towards the retromolar trigone, the buccal mucosa, the posterior portion of the floor of the mouth, and the gingiva

Tumoral spread towards superficial structures (paratonsillar region, angle of the mandible) is evaluated by determining the degree of mobility of the tonsillar region and especially by the extent of any trismus. Physical examination is basically performed to detect any cervical nodal masses in the region below the angle of the mandible.

Lymphoepithelioma of the tonsil is fairly unusual; these tumors are often polypoid and soft on physical examination, and the associated nodal masses which are almost a constant feature tend to be large and bilateral.

Overall survival at 5 years is less than 40% (Terz and Farr 1967).

6.1.3.3 Tonsillar Lymphoma

Depending on the series, tonsillar lymphoma is considered the first or second most frequent site of lymphoma in Waldeyer's ring (after the nasal and sinus cavities). The presenting symptoms are the same as for squamous cell carcinoma. The tumor generally presents as a diffuse enlargement of the entire tonsil, displacing the pillars. The clinical appearance is highly suggestive of the diagnosis when the tonsil is firm, but without induration or infiltration, and covered by red mucosal lesions. Involvement of the cervical nodes occurs in nearly all cases, and is usually bilateral.

The prognosis for tonsillar lymphoma is better than that for squamous cell carcinoma of the tonsils (Bruneton et al. 1986a).

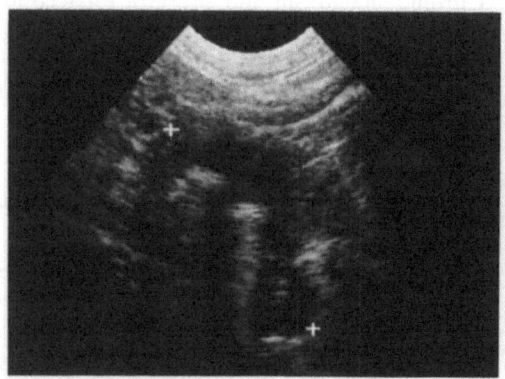

 Fig. 6.5. Cancer of the tonsil invading the glossotonsillar sulcus (38 mm between the two *crosses*)

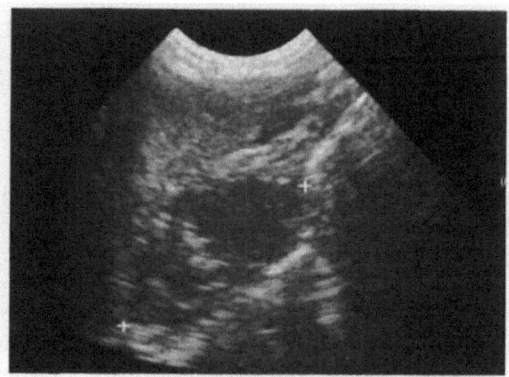

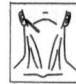 **Fig. 6.7.** Nontumoral enlargement of the tonsil in a 7-year-old child. This example is a reminder that the sonographic pattern is not specific for an etiology

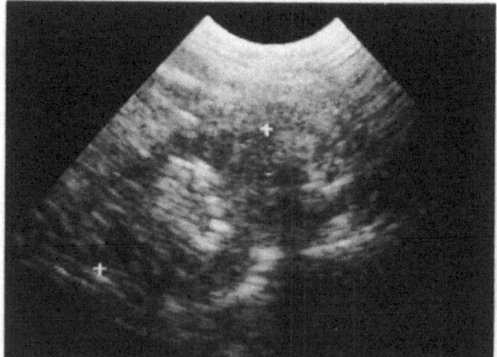

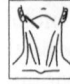 **Fig. 6.6.** Ulcerating cancer of the tonsil (33 mm between the two *crosses*); the central hyperechogenic image corresponds to an ulceration containing mucosal debris and air

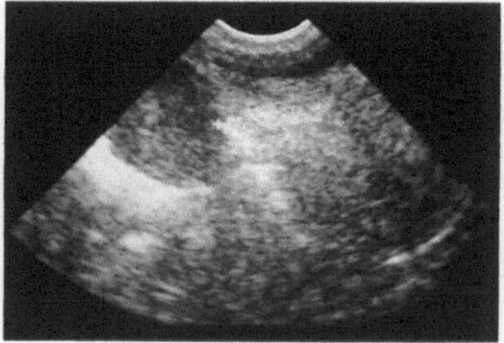

 Fig. 6.8. Non-Hodgkin's lymphoma of the tonsil (26 mm between the two *crosses*); the tongue seen anteriorly has a normal appearance

6.1.3.4 Ultrasonography of Tonsillar Lesions

Regardless of the histologic form of malignancy, tonsillar lesions can be recognized by their decreased echogenicity relative to adjacent structures. Both the diameter and margins (sharply or ill defined) must be determined. US allows satisfactory analysis of spread to the base of the tongue, and is even more sensitive than physical examination for this purpose. By contrast, neither superior nor posterior spread can be assessed sonographically (Figs. 6.5–6.8). Tumoral extension towards the paratonsillar region generally occurs only with very large tumors, and can be evaluated by US.

Whatever the histology, exploration of the lymph node-bearing areas of the neck is of prime importance, with US examination being particularly indicated (cf. Chap. 5).

6.1.4 Study of Speech and Swallowing

Shawker et al. (1985) have reported that ultrasonography is useful for the analysis of speech and swallowing, using real-time equipment and a submental approach. The tongue and the floor of the mouth are examined by sagittal, parasagittal, and coronal scans. Owing to the rapidity of movements, such studies must be recorded on videotape.

6.1.4.1 Speech Studies

The modifications of the tongue that occur during speech can be recorded, allowing measurement of the vertical displacement of the surface of the tongue and the tongue base. For Shawker et al. (1985) dynamic modifications of the tongue can be evaluated by having patients with neurologic disorders pronounce "i" and "k" sounds. Use of a radial grid system allows more accurate analysis of tongue movements. Ultrasonography has also been proposed as a biofeedback technique for speech therapy.

6.1.4.2 Swallowing

The oral phase of swallowing can be studied sonographically by videotaping the patient as he swallows a bolus of water. In normal individuals, the clearly defined muscular wave of the tongue carries the water bolus posteriorly; this oral phase is disturbed in patients with oral dysphagia (Shawker et al. 1983).

6.2 Neurogenic Tumors of the Neck

Neurogenic cervical tumors are rare lesions that can be classified into two main groups:

- tumors encountered elsewhere in the body: schwannomas, neuromas, neurofibromas, ganglioneuromas
- tumors characteristic of the cervicofacial region: esthesioneuromas, paragangliomas, gliomas, meningiomas

The most commonly encountered neurogenic tumors of the neck are schwannomas, neurofibromas (in von Recklinghausen's disease), and paragangliomas (chemodectomas) (Cernea et al. 1977).

6.2.1 Schwannomas and Neurofibromas

6.2.1.1 General Features

Schwannomas can occur at any age; they generally have a slow course and there are no spontaneous neurogenic symptoms. Schwannomas of the head and neck represent around 25% of all such tumors throughout the body. Their clinical features depend on the anatomic site. Superficial tumors may manifest as a solitary, nontender tumoral mass. Neurologic symptoms are generally not apparent unless the schwannoma develops in a narrow space rich in nerve fibers. As an example, a schwannoma in the posterior infraparotid region can cause a parapharyngeal mass with both cervical and oral clinical manifestations. Regardless of the site in the neck, a careful search must be made for neurologic involvement (especially involvement of the last four cranial nerve pairs and the cervical sympathetics). Disease recurrence is possible after ablation of a benign schwannoma, but it will also always be benign. Secondary degeneration of a benign primary schwannoma has never been reported.

Malignant schwannomas are exceedingly rare, and 75% of all such lesions occur during the course of von Recklinghausen's disease (multiple neurofibromatosis). A cervical *neurofibroma* may be the revealing symptom of a minor form of von Recklinghausen's disease. Neurofibromas may be solitary or multiple; they may arise from the superficial branches of the cervical plexus, the cranial nerves (X or XII), or the plexus cervicobrachialis.

6.2.1.2 Ultrasonography

Sonographically, small neurofibromas and schwannomas correspond to solid nodules with more or less intimate relations with the jugular and carotid vessels. The solitary nature of the lesion is the only finding suggestive of an etiology other than an adenopathy. Large tumoral masses and malignant schwannomas displace the jugular and carotid vessels as well as adjacent structures. Whereas physical ex-

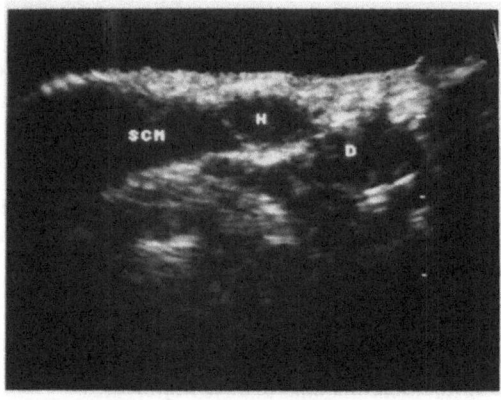

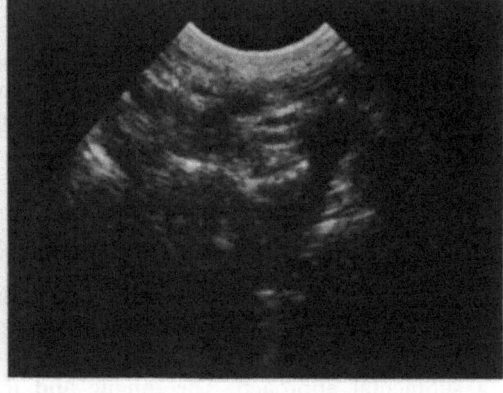

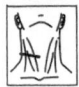
Fig. 6.9. Very superficial solid tumor between the digastric muscle *(D)* and the sternocleidomastoid muscle *(SCM)*, misdiagnosed as an enlarged node *(N)*. The surgical diagnosis was benign schwannoma

Fig. 6.11. Recurrent malignant schwannoma, with a solid, complex US pattern

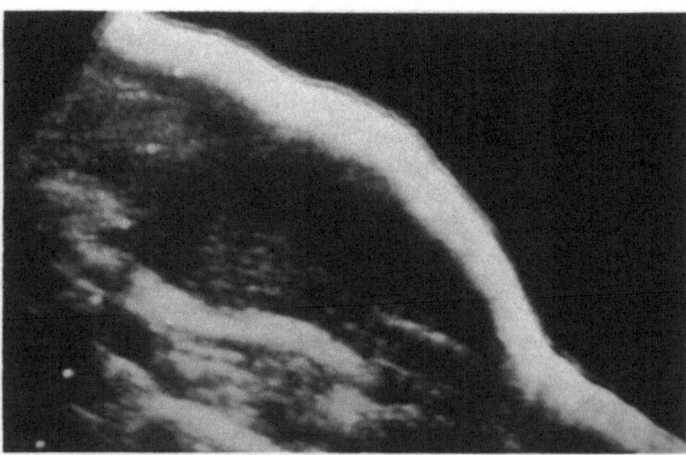

Fig. 6.10. Benign cervical schwannoma (5 cm in diameter)

amination may suggest a nodal etiology for a solitary, generally large tumoral syndrome, US will exclude this possibility. None of the information obtainable sonographically for either small focal lesions or large, obviously neoplastic masses suffices for diagnosis of a neurogenic tumor (Figs. 6.9–6.11).

6.2.2 Paraganglioma

Forms accessible for US study occur at the level of the carotid artery and the vagus nerve. Mean patient age is between 40 and 50 years; there is no marked sex predominance (Irons et al. 1977; Lack et al. 1977). These extremely rare tumors are generally benign; local recurrence is possible. Less than 10% of cases are malignant and are apt to metastasize to nodes and viscera (Bock 1982; Farr 1972; Lachard et al. 1984).

Carotid body tumors usually present as a firm, nontender mass in the lateral neck, varying in size from 2 to 10 mm. These tumors grow slowly, and neurologic signs caused by compression (dysphonia, cough, ear pain) are of late onset. Owing to the marked vascularization of these lesions, aspiration biopsy, whether performed percutaneously or surgically, is ultimately a source of diagnostic and therapeutic problems, not to mention the risk of bleeding that is hard to control. Sonographic visualization of a tumoral mass opposite the carotid bifurcation supports a diagnosis of chemodectoma (Fig. 6.12).

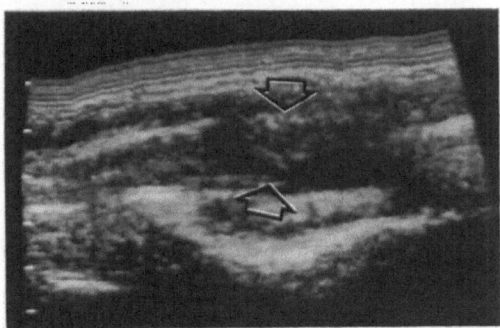

Fig. 6.12. Paraganglioma (2 cm between the *arrows*) between the internal and external carotid arteries

6.2.2.1 Ultrasonography

In practice, the value of ultrasonography appears limited when compared to three other techniques:

- Pulsed Doppler ultrasound allows detection of arterial compression, often associated with very high blood flow velocities and turbulence between the two carotid branches
- CT can evaluate tumoral hypervascularization thanks to use of intravenous contrast material; the tumor's blood supply and location orient later staging examinations
- arteriography is the most essential examination; a carotid chemodectoma is typically imaged as a very dense, finely vascularized mass; the exact relations of the tumor with the carotid and its dividing branches are accurately detailed for pretherapy purposes, and presurgical embolization may prove feasible.

Sonographic findings alone are insufficient for conclusive diagnosis of these rare cervical neurogenic tumors. US can, however, demonstrate the habitually solitary nature of such tumors, and the technique is more sensitive than physical examination. Likewise, sonographic visualization of the extension of a lesion judged superficial by physical examination (dumbbell tumor) should prompt further investigation by CT.

6.3 Cervical Cysts

Along with thyroglossal duct cysts, which account for the majority of cystic lesions in the neck apart from those in solid organs, this section describes branchial cysts, cystic lymphangioma, and dermoid cysts (Som et al. 1985).

6.3.1 Thyroglossal Duct Cysts

Thyroglossal duct cysts are the most common nonodontogenic cyst in the neck, and probably originate from the epithelial remnants of the thyroglossal tract.

6.3.1.1 General Features

During the embryonal period, the thyroid follows the descent of the heart and the great vessels; as it migrates downward, the thyroid leaves behind an epithelial trace referred to as the thyroglossal duct, which usually atrophies between the fifth and the tenth week. The caudal attachment of this duct may persist as the pyramidal lobe of the thyroid. In his review of 2284 cases of thyroglossal duct cysts, Allard (1982) found no sex predominance. Over 30% of cases are diagnosed before the patient reaches 10 years of age and only 35% of cases are not detected until the patient is 30 years or older.

Fistulae represent a potential complication of thyroglossal duct cysts, and are almost always the result of infection or trauma, occasionally of an iatrogenic nature (surgical drainage for example).

The anatomic site of the cyst habitually suggests the diagnosis, for over 75% lie in the midline of the neck; only 10%–24% are located laterally (Ward et al. 1949). Between 60% and 80% of all thyroglossal duct cysts occur below the level of the hyoid bone. Apart from those cases complicated by a fistula, the most common clinical feature is a nontender, fluctuant mass. At surgery, thyroglossal duct cysts may contain a mucoid, gelatinous, or purulent fluid. *The differential diagnoses* include branchial cysts, which are usually located more laterally, and dermoid cysts.

Carcinomatous change in a thyroglossal duct cyst occurs in approximately 1% of cases; carcinoma is almost never suspected prior to pathologic examination of the surgical specimen (Roses et al. 1983). Of such cases 80% are papillary adenocarcinomas (a frequency similar to that in thyroid cancers). Cancers of this type rarely metastasize. According to Jaques et al. (1970) the prognosis is excellent, as none of their patients died from carcinoma of a thyroglossal duct cyst.

6.3.1.2 Ultrasonography

Midline, infrahyoid thyroglossal duct cysts are generally diagnosed clinically. US merely completes the physical examination, and usually

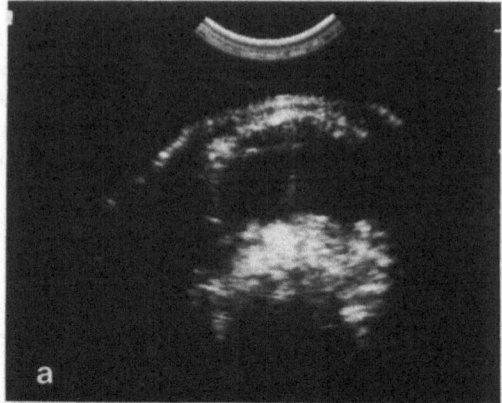
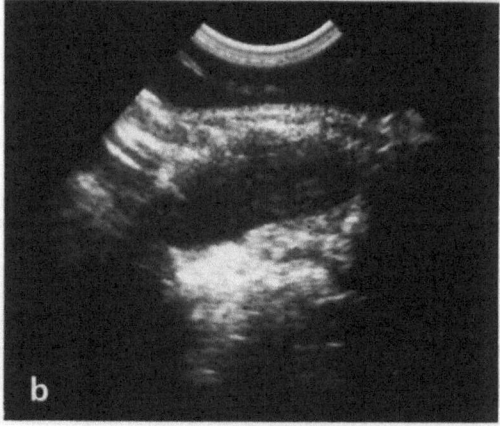
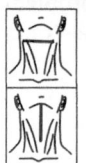

Fig. 6.13 a, b. Thyroglossal duct cyst: **a** transverse scan, **b** sagittal scan

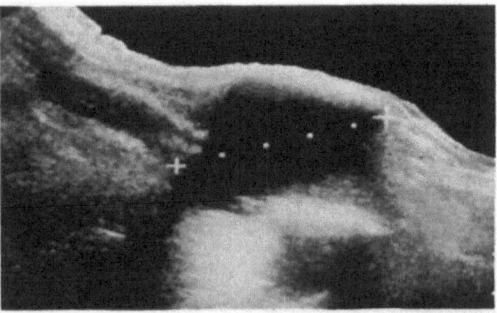

Fig. 6.14. Typical midline thyroglossal duct cyst

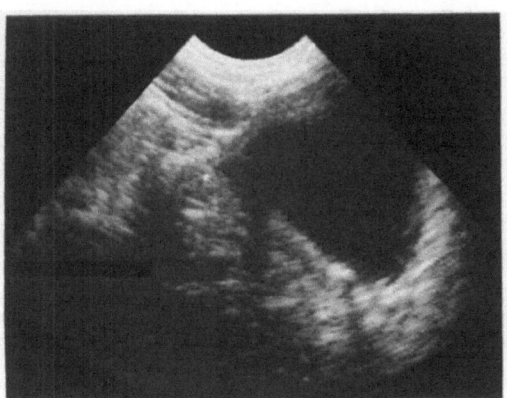

Fig. 6.15. Atypical lateral site of a thyroglossal duct cyst; US diagnosed a branchial cyst

depicts a smooth, well-limited, anechogenic mass (Figs. 6.13–6.15). It can only demonstrate the cystic nature of thyroglossal duct cysts high in the neck and in lateral sites. Regardless of the location, such findings should discourage drainage by puncture without any associated surgery because such procedures almost inevitably lead to the formation of fistulae.

6.3.2 Branchial Cyst

Most branchial cysts arise from the second branchial cleft.

6.3.2.1 General Features

Branchial cysts can be classified into four categories depending on their location: superficial cysts anterior to the sternocleidomastoid muscle, cysts lying below the middle cervical fascia and anterior to the great vessels (most frequent type), branchial extensions towards the pharynx, and intravascular cysts located between the carotid arteries and the lateral pharyngeal wall. They are most often discovered in young adults between the ages of 15 and 40 years; there is no predominance by sex and apparently no hereditary factor.

Clinically, branchial cysts present as a cervical swelling that appears rapidly over a period of several days. They tend to develop in the upper

regions of the neck, generally near the anterior belly of the sternocleidomastoid muscle, at the level of the hyoid bone. These tense, fluctuant cervical masses are painless, and the diagnosis can usually be made after physical examination. Less often, the diagnosis is suggested by a history of a recurring inflammatory neck mass, always at the same location.

The possibility of branchial cyst degeneration is still questioned and can only be proven by precise anatomic and clinical findings (MacCarthy and Turnbull 1981).

6.3.2.2 Ultrasonography

As for thyroglossal duct cysts, ultrasonography can usually only confirm the diagnosis of a branchial cyst; the lesion is generally superficial, well-limited, and anechogenic, and is located at a distance from vascular structures and the cervical organs (Figs. 6.16 and 6.17).

6.3.3 Cystic Lymphangioma

Nearly 90% of cystic lymphangiomas are detected in children before the age of 2 years. However, there have been several rare reports of diagnosis in adults between 40 and 50 years of age (Batsakis 1979; Karmody et al. 1982). These congenital malformations usually manifest as tender tumoral masses in the lateral neck; mediastinal extension is a rare possibility. The US appearance of these lesions (an anechogenic image in the lateral neck) is identical to that of branchial cysts (Fig. 6.18).

6.3.4 Dermoid Cyst

Usually located at or near the midline, a dermoid cyst is the result of epidermal inclusion during fusion of the branchial arches. The site of predilection is the hyoid region (Katz 1974). The sonographic appearance of the thick fluid often present in dermoid cysts suggests a diagnosis other than a thyroglossal duct cyst, a lesion that occurs in the same location and more frequently (Fig. 6.19).

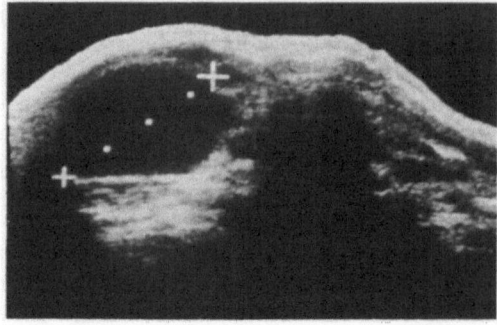

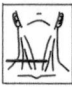
Fig. 6.16. Branchial cyst (4 cm) that developed rapidly and was considered a thyroid cyst prior to US

6.4 Spread of Local Regional Cancers

Even if physical examination suggests the origin of a large cervical tumor, ultrasound can often easily rule out certain organs as possible causes, thereby directing paraclinical exploration towards other regions. This is the case, for example, with large laryngeal and esophageal tumors that can have significant repercussions in the lateral neck when they displace the thyroid gland, the jugulocarotid vessels (with or

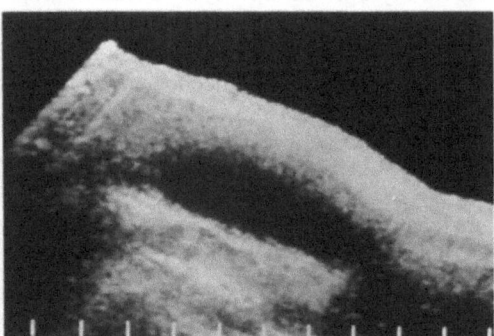

Fig. 6.17. Branchial cyst (4.5 cm)

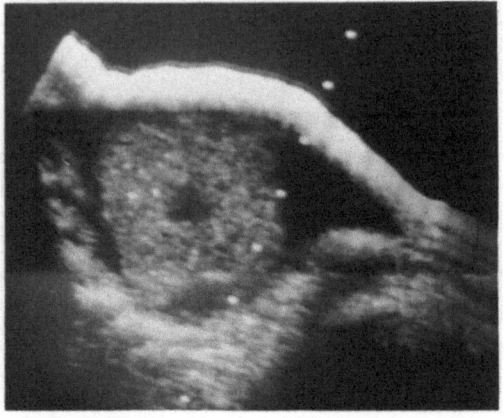

Fig. 6.19. Typical solid, midline dermoid cyst

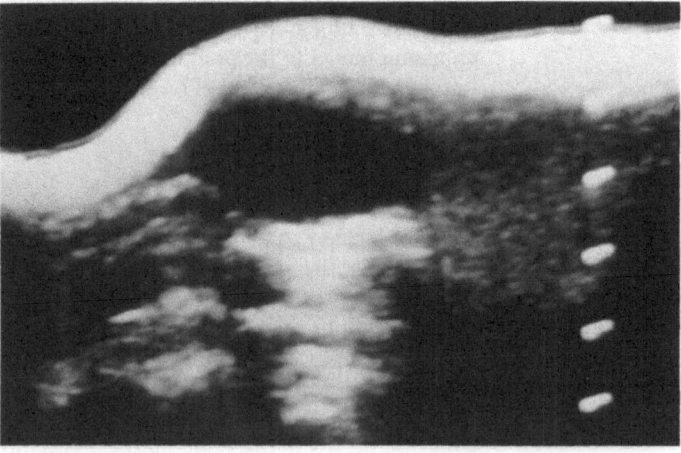

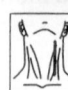
Fig. 6.18. Cystic lymphangioma considered a branchial cyst prior to surgery because of its location in the lateral neck

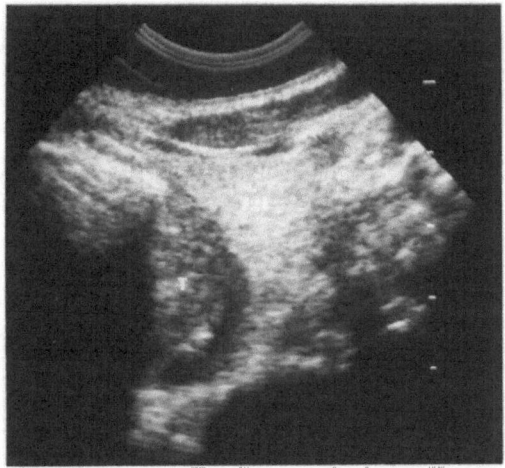

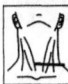 **Fig. 6.20.** Cancer of the larynx *(T)* displacing the left thyroid lobe *(TH)* laterally

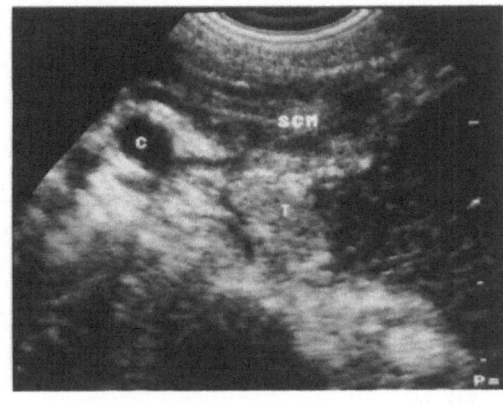

 Fig. 6.22. Postlaryngectomy abscess displacing the right thyroid lobe *(T)* laterally. *SCM*, sternocleidomastoid muscle; *C*, carotid artery

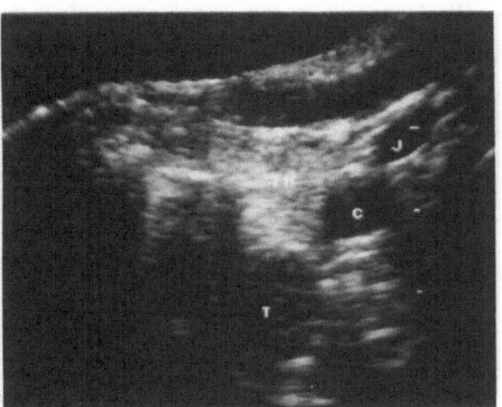

 Fig. 6.21. Cancer of the esophagus *(T)* discretely displacing the left thyroid lobe *(TH)* anteriorly. *C*, carotid artery; *J*, internal jugular vein

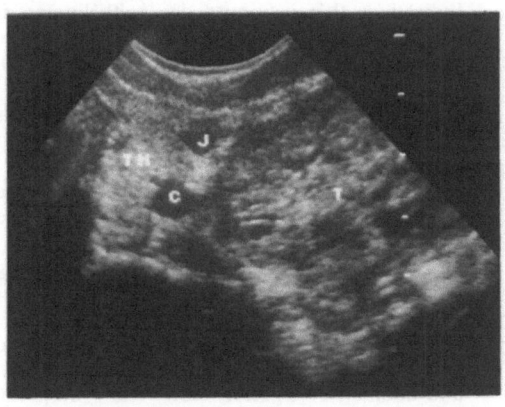

 Fig. 6.23. Thymoma *(T)* manifesting clinically as a mass in the left side of the neck displacing the lateral neck vessels medially. *TH*, thyroid gland; *J*, internal jugular vein; *C*, carotid artery

without metastatic nodes), and the lateral muscles of the neck (Figs. 6.20–6.22). Less frequently, a mediastinal tumor may manifest clinically as a cervical mass (Mikal 1974). Ultrasonography can define the upper limits of such masses and their relations with the cervical structures, while simultaneously demonstrating the absence of- a lower tumoral limit caudad (Fig. 6.23). In practice, however, US exploration of large cervical or mediastinal tumors is primarily concerned with detecting any disease spread in the neck.

6.5 References

Allard RHB (1982) The thyroglossal cyst. Head Neck Surg 5: 134–146

Apter AJ, Levine MS, Glick SN (1984) Carcinomas of the base of the tongue: diagnosis using double-contrast radiography of the pharynx. Radiology 151: 123–126

Batsakis JG (1979) Tumors of head and neck: clinical and pathological considerations, 2nd series. Williams and Wilkins, Baltimore, pp 301–304

Bock P (1982) The paraganglia. Springer, Berlin Heidelberg New York

Bruneton JN, Kerboul P, Denis F (1986a) Lymphomas of the face and neck. In: Bruneton JN, Schneider M (eds) Radiology of lymphomas. Springer, Berlin Heidelberg New York Tokyo, pp 31–39

Bruneton JN, Roux P, Caramella E, Manzino JJ, Vallicioni J, Demard F (1986b) Ultrasonography of cancer of the tongue and tonsil. Radiology 158: 743–746

Cernea P, Brocheriou C, Guilbert F, Vaillant JM, Szpirglas H, Bertrand JC, Piade R, Barrelier P (1977) Schwannomes cervico-faciaux. In: Leroux-Robert J (ed) Tumeurs nerveuses ORL et cervico-faciales. Masson, Paris, pp 85–92

Decroix Y, Ghossein NA (1981) Experience of the Curie Institute in treatment of cancer of the mobile tongue. Cancer 47: 496–508

Dulac GL, Bataini JP, Durand JC, Poncet P (1975) Indications thérapeutiques des épithéliomas du plancher buccal. In: Cernea P (ed) Les cancers du plancher de la bouche. Masson, Paris, pp 100–107

Farr HW (1972) Carotid body tumors. Thirty years' experience at the Memorial Hospital. Laryngoscope 82: 104–125

Frazell EL, Lucas JL (1962) Cancer of the tongue: report of the management of 1554 patients. Cancer 15: 1085–1099

Irons GB, Weiland LH, Brown WL (1977) Paragangliomas of the neck: clinical and pathologic analysis of 116 cases. Surg Clin North Am 57: 575–783

Jaques DA, Chambers RG, Oertel JE (1970) Thyroglossal tract carcinoma: a review of the literature and addition of eighteen cases. Am J Surg 120: 439–446

Karmody CS, Fortson JK, Calcaterra VE (1982) Lymphangiomas of the head and neck in adults. Otolaryngol Head Neck Surg 9: 283–288

Katz AD (1974) Midline dermoid tumors of the neck. Arch Surg 109: 822–823

Lachard A, Hassoun J, Charpin C, Toga M (1984) Les paragangliomes de la tête et du cou (chémodectomes). Aspects anatomo-pathologiques. In: Leroux-Robert J, Pech A (eds) Les chémodectomes (paragangliomes) cervico-céphaliques. Masson, Paris, pp 3–16

Lack EE, Cubilla AL, Woodruff JM, Farr HW (1977) Paragangliomas of the head and neck region. A clinical study of 69 patients. Cancer 39: 397–409

Larsson SG, Mancuso A, Hanafee W (1982) Computed tomography of the tongue and floor of the mouth. Radiology 143: 493–500

MacCarthy SA, Turnbull FM (1981) The controversy of bronchogenic carcinoma. Arch Otolaryngol 107: 570–572

Mikal S (1974) Cervical thymic cyst. Arch Surg 109: 558–562

Pierquin B, Chassagne D, Cachin Y, Baillet F, Fournelle Le Buis F (1970) Carcinomes épidermoïdes de la langue mobile et du plancher buccal. Etude de 245 cas traités à l'Institut Gustave Roussy. Acta Radiol (Ther) 9: 465–480

Richard J, Chassagne D, Chenal C (1975) Epithéliomas du plancher buccal antérieur sans atteinte osseuse radiologique (à propos de 97 cas). In: Cernea P (ed) Les cancers du plancher de la bouche, Masson, Paris, pp 5–14

Roses DF, Snively SL, Phelps RG, Cohen N, Blum M (1983) Carcinoma of the thyroglossal duct. Am J Surg 145: 266–269

Shawker TH, Sonies BC, Stone M, Baum BJ (1983) Real-time ultrasound visualization of tongue movement during swallowing. J Clin Ultrasound 11: 485–490

Shawker TH, Sonies B, Stone M, Garra B (1985) Ultrasound examination of speech and swallowing. J Ultrasound Med 4: 155

Som PM, Sacher M, Lanzieri CF, Solodnik P, Cohen BA, Reede DL, Bergeron RT, Biller HF (1985) Parenchymal cysts of the lower neck. Radiology 157: 399–406

Strong EW (1979) Carcinoma of the tongue. Otolaryngol Clin North Am 12: 107–114

Terz JJ, Farr HW (1967) Carcinoma of the tonsillar fossa. Surg Gynecol Obstet 125: 581–590

Vandenbrouck C, Gerard-Marchant R, Micheau C, Pierquin B, Cachin Y (1970) L'envahissement ganglionnaire des épithéliomas de la langue mobile et du plancher buccal. A propos de 367 cas traités à l'Institut Gustave Roussy de 1960 à 1965. Ann Otolaryngol 87: 779–790

Vermund H, Brennhord IO, Kaalhus O, Poppe E (1984) Squamous-cell carcinoma of the tongue: preoperative interstitial radium and external irradiation. Part II: survival. Radiology 151: 505–508

Ward GE, Hendrick JW, Chambers RG (1949) Thyroglossal tract abnormalities, cysts and fistulas. Surg Gynecol Obstet 89: 727–734

Whitaker CA, Lehr HB, Askovitz SI (1972) Cancer of the tongue. Results of treatment in 258 cases. Plastic Reconstr Surg 50: 363–370

7 Cervical Pathologies in Children

G. KALIFA, J. PONCIN, AND N. SELLIER

Exploration of the thyroid gland and the diagnosis of neck masses constitute the two major indications for cervical ultrasound in children.

7.1 Ultrasonographic Examination Technique

The technique for ultrasonographic (US) examination of the neck is the same in children as in adults. The head is slightly hyperextended by placing a pad under the shoulders. Longitudinal and transverse scans are obtained whenever possible with a 7.5 MHz transducer, although satisfactory results can also be obtained with a 5 MHz transducer in conjunction with a water bath. Real-time studies are generally preferable and, just as for adults, the sonographer must be familiar with gain adjustment, especially for the diagnosis of cysts.

The thyroid gland is the major anatomic structure seen, and both echogenically homogeneous lobes are easily visualized (Fig. 7.1). Lobe thickness varies from 8 mm at birth to 15–20 mm in young adults. The isthmus is difficult to visualize as this thin structure lies anterior to the trachea. The parathyroid glands are also hard to localize in children; only those larger than 5 mm are usually considered pathological.

7.2 Thyroid Pathologies

The anatomic information provided by ultrasonography complements that obtained with scintigraphy, and ultrasound studies have proved particularly valuable for the evaluation of thyroid dysfunction (especially hypothyroidism) and thyroid nodules.

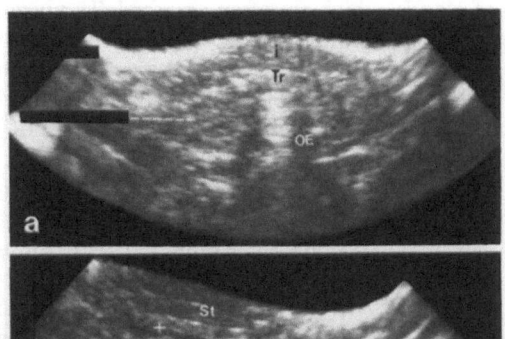

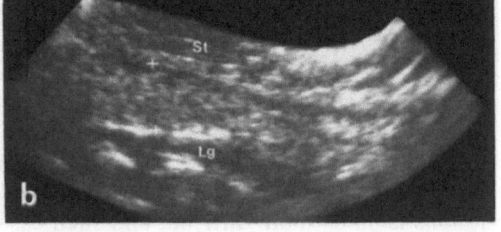

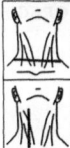

Fig. 7.1 a, b. Normal anatomy of the thyroid gland. a Transverse scan; *i*, isthmus; *Tr*, trachea; *OE*, esophagus. b Longitudinal scan; *Lg*, longus colli muscle; *St*, sternocleidomastoid muscle

7.2.1 Hypothyroidism

Today, hypothyroidism is almost always diagnosed by routine tests performed at birth. Etiological classification of the causes of hypothyroidism is particularly important, not only because it aids in epidemiological analysis of the disease, but also because it affects the prognosis and therapeutic strategy. Until recently, lesions were classified by scintigraphy, generally performed with iodine-131. At present, ultrasound along with thyroglobulin assays frequently suggests the etiology (Lemaitre et al. 1985).

Review of literature data and the statistics of the Fédération Française de Dépistage de la Maladie concur as to an incidence of nearly 55% for thyroid ectopia, 30% for complete absence of the thyroid gland or athyreosis, and 15% for hypothyroidism despite a normally located thyroid gland (Bertin and Pellerin 1982; Job and Pierson 1978).

Ultrasound examination of normally located thyroid glands is totally reliable, and the findings can be confirmed by scintigraphy. US is also a more accurate means of evaluating the size of glands, which are often enlarged. The usual cause is a hormonopoietic disorder. In cases of athyreosis, the only pitfall to be avoided with US is confusion of the pharyngolaryngeal structures with a thyroid gland; careful identification of the small images related to the presence of air in the larynx and the pyriform sinuses should eliminate this cause of error.

The major problems encountered with ultrasonography involve the diagnosis of thyroid ectopia (Fig. 7.2). Once masses attain a certain size (over 8–10 mm in diameter), their location along the path of the thyroglossal duct and their slight hyperechogenicity relative to the tongue generally lead to recognition of their thyroid nature. US diagnosis of smaller ectopic lesions is much more difficult, and such cases constitute one of the major indications for scintigraphy.

The recent development of thyroglobulin tests has improved the possibilities for etiological diagnosis. Athyreosis is usually characterized by a very low thyroglobulin level whereas children with an ectopic thyroid exhibit concentrations that are above normal. In a certain number of cases, US exploration combined with thyroglobulin tests can affirm the cause of hypothyroidism, thereby occasionally obviating the need for scintigraphy. US has the added advantage of being an easily performed, noninvasive technique. Its major limitation concerns thyroid glands smaller than 8 mm, for which radionuclide imaging remains the procedure of choice.

7.2.2 Hyperthyroidism

Hyperthyroidism is much less common than hypothyroidism in children and is generally due to Graves' disease (Fig. 7.3). Toxic adenoma is much less frequent. The diagnosis is usually provided by physical examination and scintigraphy. Although US is of less value, a diffusely hypoechogenic gland is suggestive of

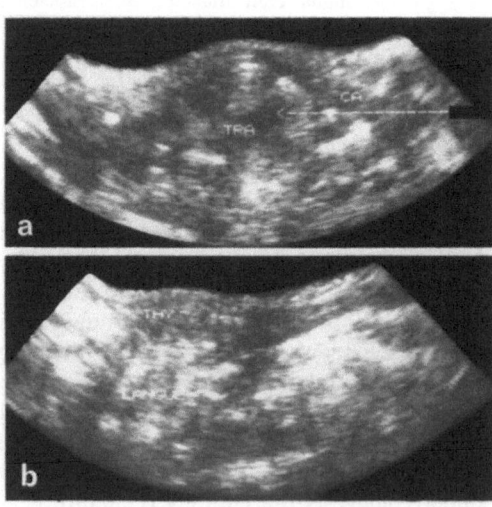

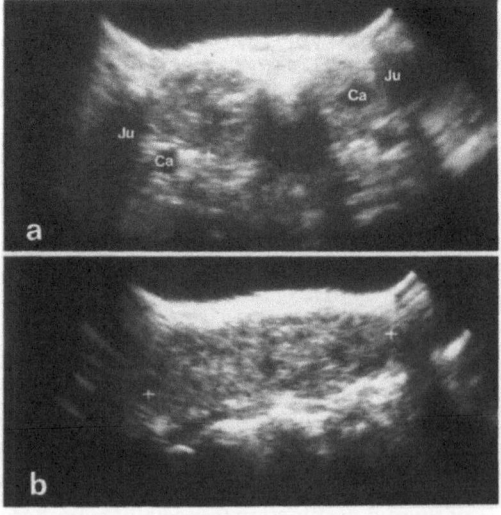

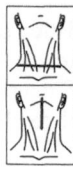

Fig. 7.2 a, b. Ectopic thyroid. **a** Transverse scan: no thyroid tissue is visible; the trachea *(TRA)* occupies most of the space next to the esophagus *(arrow)*. *CA,* common carotid artery. **b** Longitudinal scan: a midline ectopic mass is visible above the thyroid space; there is no normally located thyroid tissue

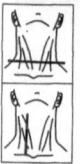

Fig. 7.3 a, b. Graves' disease. **a** Transverse scan: gland enlargement on the right displacing the vessels; complex US pattern. *Ca,* carotid artery; *Ju,* jugular vein. **b** Longitudinal scan: asymmetrical goiter in a hyperthyroid 14-year-old girl

thyroiditis while an enlarged gland of normal, homogeneous echogenicity suggests goiter.

7.2.3 Goiter and Thyroiditis

Goiter is fairly common in children. The major interest of US is detection of any malignant change (Fig. 7.4). In its early stages, goiter presents as a diffuse, more or less symmetrical, homogeneous, low density enlargement of the thyroid. With time, the internal structure is altered, resulting in more sclerous, cystic images. The main causes of goiter in children include the hormonal changes of puberty, endemic goiter, and familial disease linked to hereditary hormonogenetic disorders.

Congenital goiter may manifest as respiratory distress in a newborn; ultrasonography is an effective means of distinguishing such goiters from other causes of neck masses such as lymphangioma. In addition to hyperthyroidism in infants born of mothers with Graves' disease, goiter may occur if the mother has taken synthetic antithyroid drugs during pregnancy.

Thyroiditis is not infrequent in children (Fig. 7.5), the major cause being chronic lymphocytic thyroiditis (Hashimoto's thyroiditis). This autoimmune disease is often characterized by moderate enlargement of the gland, which is diffusely hypoechogenic. The possibility of associated nodal involvment raises the problem of differential diagnosis from lymphoma.

De Quervain's thyroiditis is rare, and can manifest as asymmetrical lobe enlargement (Fig. 7.6).

7.2.4 Thyroid Nodules

Just as in adults, thyroid nodules constitute one of the best indications for ultrasonography in children, and while such nodules are rare in young patients, they are associated with a much higher incidence of malignancy (20%–40% of all echogenic nodules in children). The three main types of lesions are pure cysts, "cold" hypofunctioning nodules, and "hot" hyperfunctioning nodules.

Thyroid cysts can be recognized by their totally anechogenic, fluidlike structure with posterior reinforcement which remains unchanged even

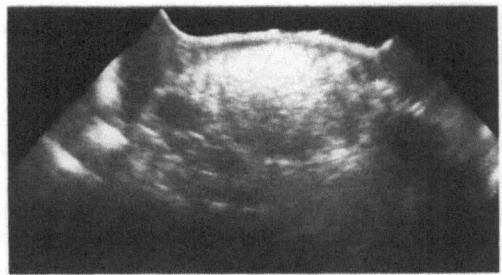

 Fig. 7.4. Multinodular goiter (longitudinal scan) with a complex US pattern; the solid component predominates, but there are hypoechogenic zones. This image is suggestive of long-standing goiter. No radionuclide uptake was observed on scintiscans obtained over several weeks

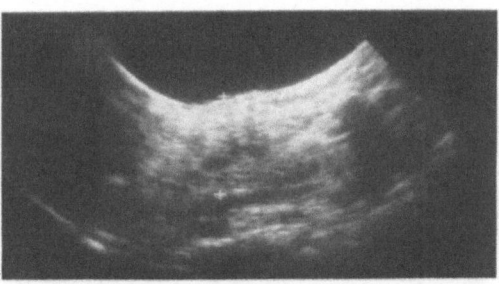

 Fig. 7.5. Infectious thyroiditis (streptococcus) (longitudinal scan): enlargement of the entire thyroid gland, with hypoechogenic zones in the medial and left portions

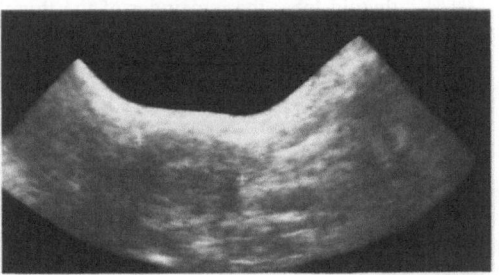

 Fig. 7.6. De Quervain's thyroiditis (longitudinal scan): enlarged, hypoechogenic left thyroid lobe; the right lobe is normal. This atypical, asymmetrical image suggests an early stage of lymphoma

at high gain settings. Such images are pathognomonic (Fig. 7.7).

Solid, hypofunctioning nodules (Fig. 7.8) carry a
high risk of malignancy. There is a marked female predominance, and neither the location,
size, consistency, nor sonographic pattern of a
nodule indicates whether it is benign or malignant. This near impossibility of differentiating
between benign and malignant lesions almost
systematically leads to immediate surgical removal. Several recent reports have described
the use of fine-needle aspiration biopsy for diagnostic purposes; in one such report, 7 of
19 nodules (36%) were found malignant in this
manner (11 adenomas, 7 carcinomas, 1 thyroiditis) (De Luca et al. 1985).

Hyperfunctioning nodules are only rarely malignant (less than 1% of cases). In a recent report
covering eight patients, only one had clinical

signs of hyperthyroidism (De Luca et al. 1986).
Nevertheless, the possibility of evolution towards severe hyperthyroidism and the slight
risk of degeneration are the basis for regular
surgical excision.

Overall, ultrasonography has a dual role in the
diagnosis of thyroid nodules. In certain cases,
US visualization of the purely fluidlike images
of cysts can obviate the need for radionuclide
scanning. Scintigraphy remains mandatory if
doubt persists as to the echogenicity of a mass,
but US examination of these patients allows a
search for associated signs (another nodule, enlarged nodes) and evaluation of gland size.
Here again, radionuclide scanning and ultrasonography are complementary, and these two
imaging techniques currently constitute the
major investigative procedures for thyroid exploration.

7.3 Neck Masses

A neck mass in a child suggests either a congenital tumor, an enlarged lymph node, or a
malignant tumor. Neoplastic processes, including both primary tumors and metastatic nodes,
account for 15% of all cervical masses in children. The main diagnostic clinical features include lesion location, the moment of appearance (a mass present at birth is considered
congenital prior to investigation), signs of malignant change if any, lesion consistency and
US pattern, lesion mobility during swallowing,
inflammation, and any distant signs. Soft
masses are especially suggestive of hemangioma or cystic lymphangioma, while a midline lesion that is mobile when the patient swallows is
suggestive of a thyroglossal duct cyst. With the
exception of thyroid cancers, most masses anterior to the sternocleidomastoid muscle are
considered benign.

7.3.1 Congenital Masses

Nearly 70% of the benign, congenital neck
masses encountered in children are thyroglossal duct cysts, 25% are branchial cysts, and
around 5% are cystic lymphangiomas (Pounds
1981).

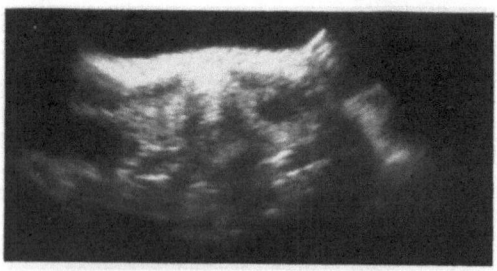

Fig. 7.7. Thyroid cyst (transverse scan):
well-limited, oval cystic structure in the left
thyroid lobe; the remainder of the thyroid
tissue is normal

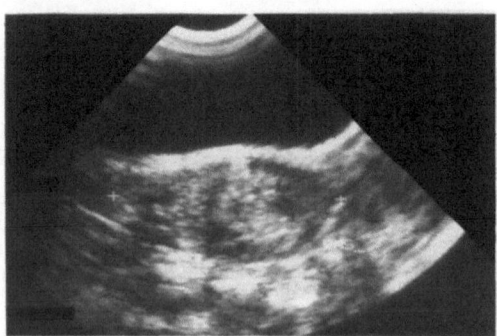

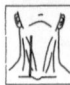
Fig. 7.8. Cold nodule in the right thyroid
lobe (longitudinal scan): nonhomogeneous
nodule of decreased echogenicity relative to
the normal adjacent thyroid tissue, surrounded by a hypoechogenic halo

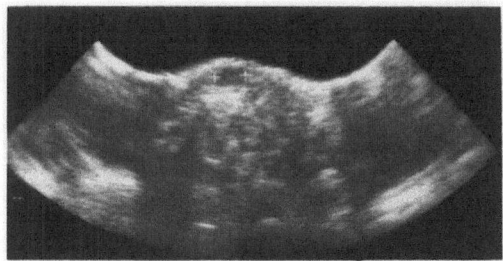

Fig. 7.9. Thyroglossal duct cyst (transverse scan): small, nonfluid hypoechogenic mass above and at a certain distance from the thyroid isthmus suggests a superinfected cyst

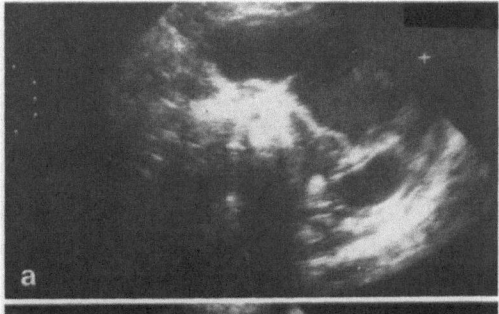

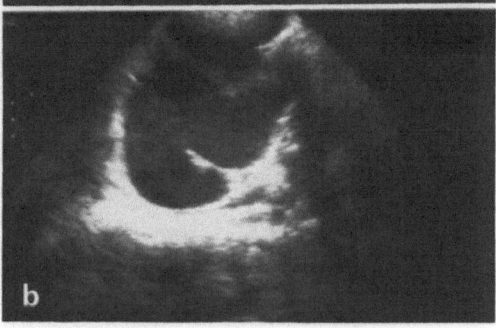

7.3.1.1 Thyroglossal Duct Cysts (Fig. 7.9)

These small midline masses located along the thyroglossal duct at the level of the hyoid bone are mobile when the patient swallows; they may be associated with fistulas. Their fluidlike nature can be demonstrated on US scans, which will also show the thyroid gland to be in its normal location. Inflammatory changes are occasionally responsible for a more complex US appearance. Thyroglossal duct cysts are usually diagnosed before the age of 5 years; the average diameter is 1–2 cm. The major differential diagnosis is a dermoid cyst, which can be mobilized with the skin and is more echogenic. Lipomas are much rarer. Care must be taken not to confuse a thyroglossal duct cyst with an ectopic thyroid gland.

7.3.1.2 Branchial Cysts

These developmental anomalies of the second branchial arch are generally not detected until later on in life. Although similar to thyroglossal duct cysts in appearance, branchial cysts differ in their location, being more lateral and anterior to the middle third of the sternocleidomastoid muscle. Branchial cysts are often associated with a cutaneous orifice. The possibility of superinfection explains the frequency of nodal involvement, but particular attention must be paid not to misdiagnose a cyst as an enlarged node. Branchial cysts require surgical removal. The branchial cleft proper is also a vestige of the third arch; the orifice is located several millimeters in front of the lower border of the ster-

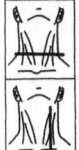

Fig. 7.10 a, b. Cystic lymphangioma. **a** Transverse scan: large, cystic mass on the left side of the neck that crosses over the midline anterior to the trachea; **b** longitudinal scan through the left side of the neck demonstrating a large cystic mass with fairly thick internal septa

nocleidomastoid muscle. Such anomalies are discovered early in life.

7.3.1.3 Cystic Lymphangioma (Figs. 7.10, 7.11)

Despite its rarity, cystic lymphangioma can occasionally be diagnosed on prenatal sonograms. These rather diffuse lesions tend to lie in a cervicomediastinal location rather than completely within the neck. Nearly 60% of cases are detected before 1 year of age, and 90% before 2 years. The unpredictable course of cystic lymphangioma can include inflammatory episodes or spontaneous involution. The mass is often located posterior to the sternocleidomastoid muscle, in the supraclavicular fossa. These cystic masses have a highly variable sonographic pattern. Lesions typically consist of multiple cysts separated by septa, but inflammatory changes frequently give the mass an echogenic appearance, preventing the identification of

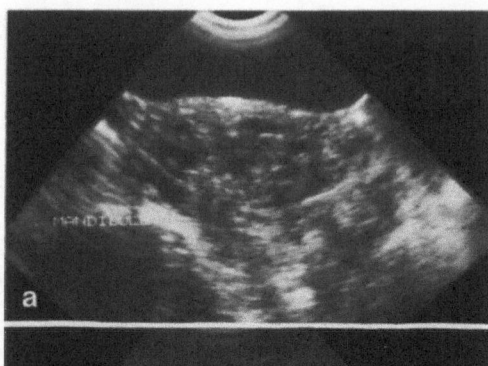

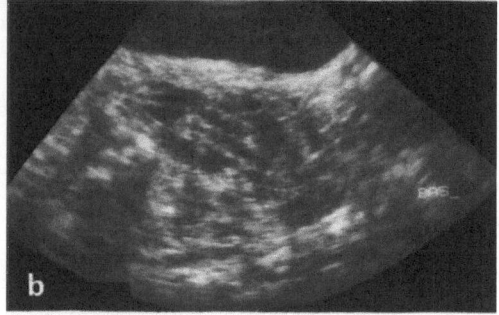

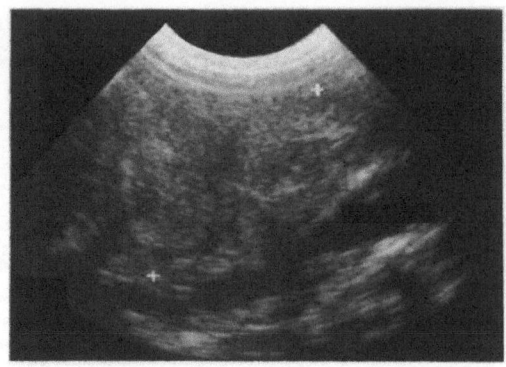

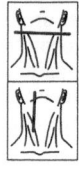

Fig.7.11a,b. Cystic lymphangioma in a 3-month-old infant: **a** transverse scan, **b** longitudinal scan. The case is similar to Fig.7.10. This large nonhomogeneous mass contains numerous hypoechogenic areas; the neck vessels (carotid artery and jugular vein) are in direct contact with the mass, which extends into the lingual sulcus *(arrow)*

Fig.7.12. Large fibrosarcoma of the neck with displacement of the carotid artery (sagittal scan: 31 mm between the two *crosses*)

7.3.1.5 Other Congenital Masses

A cervical thymus is a rare finding; the mass is mobile with respiratory movements, rising up when the child cries or during inspiration. The US pattern is solid and homogeneous. A mass in the sternocleidomastoid muscle of a newborn is especially suggestive of a hematoma.

7.3.2 Malignant Lesions

Of all neck masses in children 15% are malignant: Hodgkin's disease and non-Hodgkin's lymphomas account for 55%, rhabdomyosarcomas for 10%, and fibrosarcomas or neurofibrosarcomas for approximately 5%. The remaining lesions include thyroid cancers and neuroblastomas (Fig. 7.12).

The ultrasonographic pattern of lymphomatous lymph nodes is nonspecific. As these hypoechogenic masses tend to be multiple, a thorough search must be made for associated lesions, especially disease sites deep within the abdomen and the thorax. The possibility of leukosis or thyroid lymphoma must also be kept in mind. Imaging data for other primary tumors of the neck are not specific either; a homogeneous mass that may contain calcifications is a frequent finding. US may be sufficient for investigation of most thyroid and congenital neck masses, but malignant lesions warrant a pretherapy workup with CT to determine the extent of the disease. In addition, many of these

septa. Large cystic lymphangiomas can compress the trachea, causing respiratory distress. Such cases require CT examination after US to evaluate the extent of endothoracic spread and the exact degree of compression of the respiratory tree.

7.3.1.4 Cervical Teratomas

Cervical teratomas are rare in children. In a recent article, Gundry et al. (1983) collected 136 cases from the literature; 30 cases were associated with hydramnios, 15 infants were stillborn, and 50 of the cervical teratomas contained thyroid tissue. Respiratory distress with tracheal deviation is common, and calcifications are noted in 50% of cases. These lesions have a complex US pattern, and CT is effective for diagnosis.

masses can easily be evaluated by fine-needle aspiration biopsy.

7.4 Other Etiologies

7.4.1 Parathyroid Glands

Hyperparathyroidism is rare in children, and is usually secondary to renal insufficiency. US can detect adenomas at least 5 mm in greatest dimension. The parathyroid glands are generally imaged as oblong masses of decreased echogenicity relative to the adjacent thyroid tissue (Willi et al. 1982).

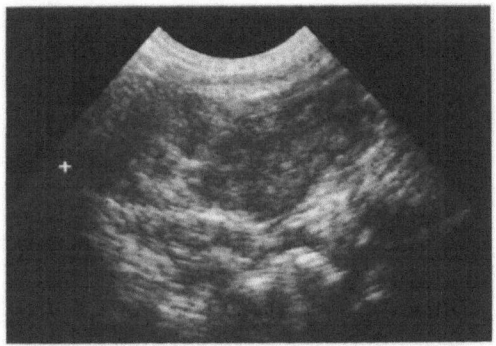

Fig. 7.13. Parotid sarcoma (6-year-old child)

7.4.2 Salivary Glands

Aside from mumps, salivary gland pathologies are uncommon in children. Submaxillary tumefaction can occur in patients with cystic fibrosis of the pancreas (mucoviscidosis) or severe malnutrition. Lithiasis of the parotid gland is exceptional in children, although there are several rare parotid tumors (Fig. 7.13).

7.5 Conclusion

To conclude, ultrasonography has considerably modified the diagnostic approach to cervical pathologies in children, and the indications for other imaging techniques are limited. Plain films are useful for evaluation of spinal lesions and diagnosis of respiratory disease and esophageal malformations (duplication). CT is generally warranted only for the workup of malignant tumors and cystic lymphangiomas. The usefulness of magnetic resonance imaging for cervical pathologies in children has not yet been demonstrated.

7.6 References

Bertin P, Pellerin D (1982) Chirurgie de la tête et du cou. In: Mozziconacci P, Saudubray JM (eds) Pédiatrie. Flammarion Médecine Science, Paris, pp 49–52

De Luca, Chaussain JL, Job JC (1985) Le nodule thyroïdien plein et hypofixant chez l'enfant et chez l'adolescent. Arch Fr Pediatr 45: 277–280

De Luca, Chaussain JL, Job JC (1986) Autonomously functioning thyroid nodules in children and adolescents. Acta Endocrinol (to be published)

Gundry S, Wesley J, Klein M, Barr M, Coran G (1983) Cervical teratomas in the newborn. J Pediatr Surg 18: 382–386

Job JC, Pierson M (1978) Endocrinologie pédiatrique et croissance. Flammarion, Paris, pp 119–180

Lemaitre L, Ythier H, Wyart D, Lemaire B, Marchandise X, Fammiaux JP (1985) Apport de l'échographie au diagnostic étiologique des hypothyroïdies congénitales. Séminaire d'Endocrinologie Pédiatrique, Paris Enfant-Malades

Pounds LA (1981) Neck masses of congenital origin. Pediatr Clin North Am 28: 841–844

Willi U, Wieland P, Rickham PP, Otto R (1982) Diagnostic ultrasonographique d'un adénome parathyroïdien et d'un calcul rénal chez une fille de 15 ans. Ann Radiol 25: 146–150

Zitelly BJ (1981) Neck masses in children. Adenopathies and malignant cells. Pediatr Clin North Am 28: 813–841